T0069776

Living with Schizophrenia

A Johns Hopkins Press Health Book ⋯⋯⋯⋯⋯⋯⋯⋯⋯⋯

LIVING
WITH
SCHIZOPHRENIA

A Family Guide to Making a Difference

JEFFREY RADO, MD, and
PHILIP G. JANICAK, MD

JOHNS HOPKINS UNIVERSITY PRESS
Baltimore

Note to the reader: This book is not meant to substitute for medical care of people with schizophrenia, and treatment should not be based solely on its contents. Instead, treatment must be developed in a dialogue between the individual and his or her physician. Our book has been written to help with that dialogue.

Drug dosage: The authors and the publisher have made reasonable efforts to determine that the selection of drugs discussed in this text conforms to the practices of the general medical community. The medications described do not necessarily have specific approval by the U.S. Food and Drug Administration for use in the diseases for which they are recommended. In view of ongoing research, changes in governmental regulation, and the constant flow of information relating to drug therapy and drug reactions, the reader is urged to check the package insert of each drug for any change in indications and dosage and for warnings and pre-cautions. This is particularly important when the recommended agent is a new and/or infrequently used drug.

© 2016 Johns Hopkins University Press
All rights reserved. Published 2016
Printed in the United States of America on acid-free paper
9 8 7 6 5 4 3 2

Johns Hopkins University Press
2715 North Charles Street
Baltimore, Maryland 21218-4363
www.press.jhu.edu

Library of Congress Cataloging-in-Publication Data

Names: Rado, Jeffrey, 1970- author. | Janicak, Philip G., author.
Title: Living with schizophrenia : a family guide to making a difference /
    Jeffrey Rado, MD, and Philip G. Janicak, MD.
Description: Baltimore : Johns Hopkins University Press, [2016] | Includes
    bibliographical references and index.
Identifiers: LCCN 2016010033| ISBN 9781421421421 (hardcover : alk. paper) |
    ISBN 1421421429 (hardcover : alk. paper) | ISBN 9781421421438 (pbk. : alk.
    paper) | ISBN 1421421437 (pbk. : alk. paper) | ISBN 9781421421445
    (electronic) | ISBN 1421421445 (electronic)
Subjects: LCSH: Schizophrenia—Popular works. | Schizophrenia—Treatment—
    Popular works. | Schizophrenia—Family relationships.
Classification: LCC RC514 .R26 2016 | DDC 616.89/8—dc23
    LC record available at https://lccn.loc.gov/2016010033

A catalog record for this book is available from the British Library.

Special discounts are available for bulk purchases of this book. For more information, please contact Special Sales at 410-516-6936 or specialsales@press.jhu.edu.

Johns Hopkins University Press uses environmentally friendly book materials, including recycled text paper that is composed of at least 30 percent post-consumer waste, whenever possible.

Contents

Preface   *vii*

1   What Is Schizophrenia?   1

2   What Causes Schizophrenia?   21

3   Biological Therapies for Schizophrenia   34

4   Psychosocial and Behavioral Treatments for Schizophrenia   55

5   Staying Well   63

6   Schizophrenia and the Family   77

7   Medical Conditions and Schizophrenia   93

Conclusion: Looking to the Future   108

Notes   *115*
Index   *121*

Preface

The idea for this book grew out of our time working with people affected by schizophrenia, a condition that is perplexing to patients and caregivers alike. Much about schizophrenia is misunderstood or poorly understood. We felt there was a need for a brief yet informative resource for those seeking to better understand this disorder—a guide that directly spoke to you, the person diagnosed with schizophrenia, and you, the family member. Our goal with this book is to present information in plain English without medical jargon; to be neither too lengthy nor too simplistic; and to convey an understanding and empathy that goes beyond a medical textbook.

When we first meet with a person who has schizophrenia and her family, we sit down together and try to help them make sense of this condition. We try to take into account their belief system, values, and cultural background. This initial conversation allows us to discover what is of most concern to the person who has schizophrenia and her family. In this way, we can better understand each other and find a mutually agreeable starting point for discussion. Ultimately, we try to convey to them the knowledge and understanding that will allow them to best achieve recovery and healing.

Between us, we have more than sixty years of experience working with individuals and their families. Philip Janicak has written more than one hundred articles, chapters, and books and given countless lectures nationally and internationally on the topic of schizophrenia. In that context, he has educated many of the psychiatrists practicing today. As a board-certified psychiatrist and internal medicine specialist, Jeffrey Rado's focus has been to improve both the mental and the physical health of persons with schizophrenia. Both of us have conducted research in the area of mental illness and more specifically on treatment approaches to schizophrenia.

How to Read This Book

The book begins, in chapter 1, by describing what schizophrenia is and what its symptoms are, including the positive and negative symptoms (characteristics that are either present or absent) and cognitive symptoms that are the core symptoms of schizophrenia, as well as changes in behavior, mood, and concentration. This chapter also includes an explanation of how a diagnosis is made. Chapter 2 explores the causes of schizophrenia, including genetics, brain changes, and environmental factors.

Chapters 3 and 4 provide detailed explanations of medications (chapter 3) and psychological treatments (chapter 4), including how treatments are modified for the different stages of schizophrenia, as well as a description of the wide variety of supportive therapies that often provide great benefit to people with schizophrenia and their families.

Chapters 5 and 6 offer practical, specific advice for persons who are diagnosed with schizophrenia (chapter 5) and for their family members (chapter 6). Chapter 5 emphasizes the importance of routine and vigilance, and chapter 6 describes how family members can best help the person with schizophrenia—and themselves.

Chapter 7 is an important discussion about how to enhance the physical health of the person with schizophrenia.

We note important points in each chapter for easy reference. Some chapters include Internet resources and other references. The book is relatively short, reflecting our goal of making it possible to read in one sitting, if the reader wishes. The chapters can be read separately, and the index makes it easy to find specific topics of interest.

Being told that you have schizophrenia can be a traumatic experience. Learning that a loved one has schizophrenia can be equally distressing. Our wish is for this book to empower you with the knowledge and awareness you need to promote wellness and to begin the healing process.

Our inspiration is you—the individuals and families coping every day with this challenging illness.

Living with Schizophrenia

1

What Is Schizophrenia?

When you, or a person close to you, were first diagnosed with schizophrenia, your first reaction might have been fear and confusion, wondering, *"How could this have happened?"* Or your overwhelming emotion might have been disbelief: *"It can't be true."* The image of a person with schizophrenia that is presented in movies and TV is often both negative and inaccurate. For instance, the individual is often portrayed as violent and unpredictable, when in fact most people who have schizophrenia are not dangerous. Despite what is commonly thought, schizophrenia does not involve "switching personalities" or "multiple personalities." Schizophrenia *is* a disabling disorder, involving abnormal brain function that alters the way people perceive the world. It affects all areas of functioning—at school, at work, and in relationships—and impairs people's ability to care for themselves.

Family members may have noticed that their relative with schizophrenia acts and thinks differently from most other people. Prominent symptoms of schizophrenia include hallucinations and delusions, changes in behavior and speech, and changes in how emotions are expressed. Additionally, people who have schizophrenia may experience changes in mood (such as depression), feel anxious, have difficulty focusing and concentrating, and make unusual movements.

If someone in the family has schizophrenia, family members are significantly affected (help for family members is offered in chapter 6). The symptoms of altered sensory experiences (that is, hearing voices, thinking that others are talking about them) are often puzzling to family members and mental health care providers alike. The illness makes it difficult for the affected person to tell the difference between what is real and what is unreal. In addition to describing these symptoms in more detail, this chapter explains how schizophrenia is diagnosed. We also review the onset of the illness, its course, and its long-term outcome.

How Schizophrenia Has Been Defined over Time

The definition of schizophrenia has evolved with advances in our understanding of this perplexing illness. One of the earliest descriptions of schizophrenia was made by the late nineteenth-century German psychiatrist Emil Kraepelin. He was the first to conceptualize it as a syndrome—a specific pattern of symptoms appearing over time—which he labeled "dementia praecox." Dementia praecox consisted of psychosis (a disconnection from reality) combined with disordered thinking (impaired memory, attention, and behavior) and social withdrawal. More than purely a collection of symptoms, this syndrome described a specific onset (adolescence or early adulthood), course (worsening over time), and outcome (described as "mental dullness") that differed from other illnesses, such as manic depression (now referred to as bipolar disorder). Kraepelin made a distinction between schizophrenia, with its prominent cognitive deficits, chronic course, and worse functioning, and bipolar disorder, with predominant mood symptoms, a waxing and waning course, and better functioning.

Nineteenth-century Swiss psychiatrist Eugen Bleuler coined the term "schizophrenia." He described mild cases of schizophrenia with relatively good outcomes, leading to the view of schizophrenia as a heterogeneous disorder, meaning it has multiple causes, whose ultimate course and outcome varies among individuals. He identified the key symptoms of affective flattening (lack of emotional expression), low motivation, and difficulties with social relationships. These were later classified as negative symptoms, that is, symptoms notable for an absence of thoughts or feelings. Bleuler also described the split in schizophrenia between perception and reality: what the person believes or experiences may not be reality based. This "split" is different from "split personality," which is a separate psychiatric disorder in which a person has two or more personalities.

In the twentieth century, psychiatrist Kurt Schneider emphasized the diagnostic importance of hallucinations and delusions such as thought withdrawal (belief that an outside force is removing thoughts), thought insertion (belief that an outside force is putting thoughts in), and thought broadcasting (belief that everyone can hear his thoughts). He also described commonly occurring auditory hallucinations consisting of the person hearing a running commentary about himself, or two voices having a conversation in the person's head.

Diagnosis of Schizophrenia

Making a diagnosis of schizophrenia can be challenging. Specific symptoms, such as hallucinations or other delusions, can certainly indicate schizophrenia. But the diagnosis is based on more than just the presence of one or two symptoms; the health care professional making the diagnosis must also consider the pattern and combination of symptoms over time. A diagnosis of schizophrenia is made only in people who have two or more of the following symptoms for at least one month during a six-month period: delusions, hallucinations, disorganized speech, disorganized or catatonic behavior, and negative symptoms. Regardless of the duration or number of symptoms, those who are diagnosed with schizophrenia have at some point had trouble at school or work, problems taking care of themselves, or difficulties in their relationships with other people. The difficulties must involve a change from a higher level of functioning in the period before the symptoms began.

Symptoms typically first become evident in men when they are in their late teens or early twenties, and in women in their late twenties. Less commonly, individuals do not experience symptoms until their thirties or forties, but rarely do symptoms appear for the first time later in life.

Positive Symptoms: Delusions and Hallucinations

Delusions and hallucinations are known as *positive symptoms*, meaning symptoms that are noteworthy for the characteristics that are present (it does not mean positive in the sense of desirable or good). Positive symptoms are a hallmark of schizophrenia. Delusions may be thought of as strongly held beliefs that are not supported by the reality of life. The perception, in fact, may have no connection to reality. Delusions are frequently manifested by odd or absurd thoughts or feelings:

> Clarence, 44 years old, has schizophrenia. He is afraid to go out of the house on most days and will not use the telephone. His mother asked him why he was whispering to her all the time. He responded, "So they won't hear me." He later explained that the government was using satellites to monitor his every movement because "they want to control my brain."

This is an example of a persecutory delusion. There is no proof that the government intends to harm Clarence, but he feels certain it is true. Delusions may be "grandiose," meaning that people think that they are special or talented in some way or that they are in a close relationship with a famous person. For instance, people with grandiose delusions may think they are famous movie stars or Jesus Christ or that their lives are a TV show or movie that everyone is watching.

> Fred is a 29-year-old who has schizophrenia. He thinks he is going to marry a famous pop star. He told his mother that he and the star have several children together and that the two were meant to be together.

People with schizophrenia may experience these other types of delusions as well:

- *Referential* (also called *idea of reference*): They feel that events or objects in the environment have special meaning for them, for example, believing that a flashing red stoplight is telling them their life is in danger, or that Facebook postings are conveying a special message just for them.
- *Erotomanic*: They believe that someone is in love with them.
- *Somatic:* The delusion is focused on their health or the functioning of their bodily organs, for example, sensing that someone or something is living in their bowels.
- *Nihilistic*: They may be convinced that a major catastrophe is going to occur, for example, believing that the end of the world, or the apocalypse, is coming.
- *Thought broadcasting*: They believe that others can hear their thoughts out loud.
- *Thought insertion*: They think that someone or something is inserting thoughts into their mind.
- *Thought withdrawal*: They believe that an outside person or force is removing thoughts from their mind.

- *Guilt*: They believe they have done something terribly wrong. This may be accompanied by a belief that they deserve to be punished for the misdeed.

Hallucinations are perceptions that are experienced as real but that are not real. These experiences are not under the person's voluntary control. For instance, a person might hear a voice telling him to bake a cake, but others in the environment do not hear the voice. The person perceives the voice as coming through his ears or inside his head, not from his own thoughts. The experience can range from clear words and sentences to indecipherable mumbling, whispering, or chatter. You may notice your loved one talking out loud to himself. This may occur when he is responding to a hallucination. Other types of hallucinations are visual (seeing things that no one else can see), tactile (the sensation of being touched), or olfactory (experiencing smells or odors). For example, some individuals describe smelling formaldehyde or "dead people."

When delusions or hallucinations become too intense or there is concern that the person may harm himself or others, hospitalization may be required. Despite treatment, up to 50 percent of all individuals with schizophrenia experience persistent positive symptoms.

Negative Symptoms

In contrast to positive symptoms, negative symptoms are notable for what is missing, specifically, the absence of thoughts or feelings. You may have noticed that your loved one has lost interest in things that she used to enjoy. Maybe she no longer talks to anyone, and she spends more time alone. She may have stopped participating in a sport or a favorite hobby. These are examples of negative symptoms. Other negative symptoms of schizophrenia are:

- Reduced facial expressions (or *blunted affect*): People may not laugh, smile, get angry, or react to situations that ordinarily would elicit a response. For example, they might describe a terrifying experience without demonstrating any fear or anxiety. Their facial expressions may be blank.
- Lack of motivation (also called *avolition* or *apathy*): They may sit alone for long periods without doing anything. They may drop out of school or stop attending to basic self-care, such as shaving and bathing.
- Decreased talking (also called *alogia* or *poverty of speech*): People may speak very little or respond with simple one-word answers. When asked a question, they may sit in silence for a long time before saying anything. This makes it difficult to engage them in even simple conversation.
- *Asociality* is a lack of interest in talking to or spending time with others. People with this symptom may avoid social gatherings, preferring instead to spend time alone in their room. *Anhedonia* is a lack of pleasure in activities that were fun in the past but that are no longer interesting or enjoyable.

Of note, people with schizophrenia may not view any of the above symptoms as problematic. They may not be bothered by their apparent lack of motivation and minimal social interaction with others.

Definitions

Psychosis: Mental state characterized by disconnection from reality. Typically associated with hallucinations and delusions.

Positive symptoms: Symptoms that are noticeable, such as delusions, hallucinations, and disordered thoughts and speech.

Delusion: A firmly held but false belief that is not based on reality.

Hallucination: Seeing or hearing things that don't exist; *perception* in the absence of external *stimulus.*

Negative symptoms: Symptoms that reflect an absence, such as lack of emotion, facial expression, motivation, and social interaction.

Disorganized Speech

People with schizophrenia may not speak in a clear manner. Not speaking clearly indicates their disorganized thinking, which may be exhibited by any of the following:

- Switching between distantly related topics (*looseness of association*).
- Not making sense or making comments that are completely unrelated to the topic being discussed (*derailment*).
- Connecting unrelated ideas in the same sentence, speaking in incomplete sentences or with words mixed up (word salad), using made-up words (neologisms), or repeating the same words over and over. The person may seem to have invented a new way of talking. This speech pattern results from disconnected thoughts.
- Veering off the topic being discussed (tangentiality) when answering questions.

As a result of disorganized speech, the affected person may have difficulty communicating with family members or health care providers. It may also make it difficult to attend school or function in work and social settings.

Disorganized Behavior

People who have schizophrenia may engage in actions that do not serve a clear purpose. For instance, they may repeatedly wring their hands, stare into the mirror for long periods, or stir a pot that has nothing in it. Some may wander aimlessly in the middle of night. They may act silly at some moments but appear restless and hyperactive at other times. People with schizophrenia may watch static on TV, spend hours arranging pebbles on the ground in a specific way, or put glue in their hair. Inappropriate giggling during serious situations (such as a funeral) can be both puzzling and disturbing to family members.

Other Symptoms

Problems with Thinking

Difficulties with mental processes (called *cognitive impairment*) are extremely common in people who have schizophrenia and tend not to improve much over time. Up to 75 percent of all patients demonstrate long-lasting impairments in thinking. In addition, these difficulties persist even when the other symptoms of schizophrenia (such as hearing voices) are under control. This is one of the main reasons that people with schizophrenia have difficulty with schoolwork, keeping a job, or managing finances. The affected areas include:

- *Attention and concentration*: The person may have difficulty staying focused on specific information and not getting distracted by other stimuli in the environment. For instance, sounds such as a car horn, a baby crying, or a dog barking may interfere with the person's ability to follow a conversation.
- *Working memory*: The person may forget what someone tells him, such as forgetting to take his medication despite every intention to do so, or forgetting appointments, people's names, or what he was supposed to pick up at the grocery store.
- *Verbal fluency and language*: The person has difficulty finding words to say. She may take a long time to respond to others in conversation.

- *Social cognition* (reacting appropriately in social situations): The person is not able to understand or respond to other peoples' emotions. He may have impaired comprehension of facial expressions or tones of voice that convey anger, fear, excitement, or other emotions.
- *Planning, reasoning, and problem solving*: The person is unable to complete complex tasks, plan appropriately, or solve problems logically. She may have difficulty working toward personal goals and grasping new concepts in school or work settings. She may have trouble managing her money; a previously learned task like balancing a checkbook may become difficult. Understanding new ideas or following the shift between different topics or ideas may be challenging.
- *Processing speed*: This refers to the speed with which a person can take in and make sense of new information. The person may process information more slowly than others, so completing tasks may require extra time. He may take a long time to respond in a conversation, and delays in response may lead to social awkwardness.

Changes in Emotions: Depression and Anxiety

Many people affected by schizophrenia experience depression or anxiety. Almost half of people with schizophrenia report symptoms of depression early in their illness. Common depression symptoms include feeling down or blue, poor sleep, hopelessness, low energy, and poor appetite. The person may appear sad, and her mood may also quickly change from happy to sad.

People with schizophrenia also frequently complain of anxiety and may report feeling nervous, worried, or on edge. Specific types of anxiety, such as *obsessive-compulsive disorder* (for example, repeated behaviors such as hand-washing while having obsessive thoughts about germs) or *agoraphobia* (fear of situations that might make a person panic), are also common. Disturbing hallucinations or delusions can cause anxiety. For instance, people who believe they are being monitored by the FBI may feel anxious whenever they venture outside the house. They may, in fact, never leave their house because of this fear.

Changes in Movements

At times people who have schizophrenia may adopt rigid and seemingly bizarre postures. They might not speak or move at all (called *mutism*). Some make faces, blink repetitively, stare intensely, or exhibit various mannerisms, such as repeatedly turning their head or raising their eyebrows. They might make gestures with their hands or limbs, rock back and forth in their seats, or move their entire bodies. Some people with schizophrenia imitate or repeat the movements of others (*echopraxia*). Movements may be clumsy and awkward. *Catatonic behavior* may take several forms:

- Remaining in an odd or rigid posture for long periods
- Resisting others' attempts to move their limbs or make them walk
- Engaging in constant activity without any purpose

Initial Evaluation

The diagnosis of schizophrenia is made by a medical doctor specializing in the diagnosis and treatment of mental illness (a psychiatrist) or by another mental health professional (such as a psychologist). You may get a referral to a psychiatrist from your primary care doctor, through your health care insurance, or by contacting the National Alliance on Mental Illness (NAMI) or the American Psychiatric Association (APA).

The psychiatric diagnosis is based on an interview with the individual as well as with a family member, and sometimes others who know the person well. The provider asks what the symptoms are, how long the person has been experiencing them, and the possible role of drugs, alcohol, or other factors that might be important. The purpose of the interview is to assess whether the person has symptoms that fit the diagnostic criteria, such as hallucinations, delusions, and reduced expression of emotions. The diagnostic criteria are described in the fifth edition of the *Diagnostic and Statistical Manual of Mental Disorders*, fifth edition, Text Revision *(DSM-5-TR)*. The *DSM-5-TR* is a book written by experts in the field of psychiatry, published by the American Psychiatric Association, the largest professional organization of psychiatrists in the United States.

The person does not have to experience all the described symptoms all the time to be diagnosed with schizophrenia. You have probably noticed that your loved one has some really good days when she interacts quite well and thinks more clearly, but then on other days, her mood may change or she may talk out loud when no one is there, as if she were responding to someone or something that no one else can see or hear. This is typical of how schizophrenia affects people, even those who take their medication regularly. Most people with schizophrenia experience some problems with work, school, or social relationships, so the provider will assess how the individual has been functioning in these areas over the long run.

Symptoms change and evolve over time, which means that different diagnoses are sometimes made in the same person at different points in time. Your loved one may have initially been given other diagnoses. For instance, in the early stages of the illness, a teenager may not talk much and prefer to spend a lot of time alone in his room. This "moodiness" may initially be attributed to "being a teenager." Later, the individual may start to ignore his personal appearance, say things that you consider to be odd, and withdraw from those around him. As these other symptoms develop, the diagnosis may be changed to schizophrenia. Depression is common in schizophrenia, and many of the negative symptoms of schizophrenia (such as lack of pleasure and avoiding social interaction) resemble depression. As a result, depression is sometimes initially diagnosed when the more appropriate diagnosis is schizophrenia. This is one of several reasons that it is important to continue treatment with a mental health care provider, to receive the most comprehensive assessment possible.

No blood tests, x-rays, CT scans, or MRI tests can diagnose schizophrenia. Mental health care providers use information such as age of onset, symptoms, and relationship of the symptoms to possible triggering events in order to judge whether a more extensive medical evaluation is necessary. The initial evaluation of any person with psychotic symptoms must consider causes of psychosis other than schizophrenia. A thorough medical history and a physical examination may be called for in someone being newly evaluated for psychosis, to evaluate for medical causes of these symptoms, such as an infection, a brain injury, a brain tumor, or another medical cause.

Before becoming ill, people who later develop schizophrenia are often typical of other young adults of the same age. They may have done well in school, had a lot of friends, or played on the high school basketball team. A significant and stressful event may trigger the appearance of symptoms, such as a difficult breakup, the death of someone close, or starting college and becoming overwhelmed by the academic demands. Sometimes there is no trigger. The role of stress and other factors are more fully discussed in chapter 2.

Schizophrenia-Spectrum Disorders

Although schizophrenia is the most common psychotic disorder, several separate but related disorders may resemble schizophrenia. In other words, having psychotic symptoms does not automatically mean a person has schizophrenia. These other disorders, called schizophrenia-spectrum disorders, include schizophreniform disorder, brief psychotic disorder, schizoaffective disorder, delusional disorder, schizotypal personality disorder, schizoid personality disorder, and paranoid personality disorder. All of these conditions have similar symptoms and treatments.

People with schizophreniform disorder have the same symptoms as people with schizophrenia, though the total duration of symptoms is less than six months, and people with schizophreniform disorder maintain normal functioning. Brief psychotic disorder describes psychosis that may be brought on by severe stress but that resolves completely within one month of onset.

Schizoaffective disorder involves the same symptom criteria as schizophrenia, with one exception: mood symptoms (significant depression or mania) are present a majority of the time. There must be at least a two-week period when the person has psychosis but no mood symptoms. Mood symptoms may involve depressed mood or elevated or angry mood (as seen in bipolar disorder). Differentiating schizophrenia from schizoaffective disorder can be challenging because (1) the negative symptoms of schizophrenia may resemble depression, and (2) it can be difficult to confirm how long mood symptoms last and whether they are present for a "majority" of the time.

Delusions are the only psychotic symptom in people who are diagnosed with delusional disorder. In general, these individuals do not experience hallucinations, negative symptoms, or disorganized speech or behavior. Although social or occupational problems may result, functioning is not impaired to the degree seen in schizophrenia, and behavior is not bizarre or odd.

Schizotypal personality disorder is characterized by persistent and widespread impairments in social and interpersonal functioning, such as decreased ability to form intimate relationships and eccentric or odd behavior, thinking, or appearance. People may talk about bizarre ideas and perceptions, report suspiciousness or paranoid ideas, or be preoccupied with mental telepathy or magical beliefs. Symptoms are milder, and those with this disorder are generally not hospitalized. Schizotypal personality disorder usually becomes evident in early adulthood but sometimes appears in adolescence. Abnormalities of beliefs, thinking, and perception are not distorted to the degree that they are with schizophrenia.

People with schizoid personality disorder tend to be socially isolated, spending most of their time alone and not having any friends. They appear to be indifferent to others—lacking any emotion or sense of connection with others.

Paranoid personality disorder describes people who pervasively feel that the world is against them. They feel easily slighted by others, are suspicious of others' motivations, and think others are trying to deceive them.

Disorders That May Be Confused with Schizophrenia

Just as schizophrenia can be mistaken for another disorder, several psychiatric disorders, including bipolar disorder and major depression, can initially be mistaken for schizophrenia. The symptoms of depression and bipolar disorder overlap with those of schizophrenia. As a result, people with schizophrenia at some point may be misdiagnosed as having a mood disorder. If psychotic symptoms occur only when mood symptoms are present, then the correct diagnosis may be a mood disorder. Bipolar disorder is a mood disorder that involves periods of intense and irritable or elevated moods (*mania*) alternating with feelings of low or depressed moods. Major depression is a mood disorder characterized primarily by periods of low or sad feelings. Depressed persons may also speak less, show less emotion, and isolate themselves from others. These behaviors may resemble the negative symptoms of schizophrenia.

When people who have a mood disorder are experiencing symptoms of that disorder, they may experience psychotic symptoms when their mood symptoms are more intense. For instance, a person experiencing mania may have grandiose delusions, thinking he has super powers or special talents, or that he is famous. Alternatively, a depressed person may hear voices telling her that she is worthless or that she should do harm to herself. In both cases, symptoms resemble schizophrenia but are primarily a manifestation of a mood disorder. In contrast, persistent psychosis that occurs without any mood symptoms (such as sadness, anger, or elevated mood) is more likely to be a sign of schizophrenia. People with mood disorders also tend to function better in school, work, and relationships than people with schizophrenia, who are frequently unable to attend school or hold a job. Last, schizophrenia tends to begin earlier in life than major depression or bipolar disorder.

People with obsessive-compulsive disorder have strong beliefs (called obsessions) that are relieved by performing certain rituals (called compulsions). For instance, someone extremely worried about germs may wash his hands incessantly. People with obsessive-compulsive disorder may lack insight and be completely persuaded that their obsessive-compulsive beliefs are true. The diagnosis would be obsessive-compulsive disorder with poor insight. Similarly, individuals with body dysmorphic disorder may be completely convinced that there is something deformed or abnormal about their body. Although this may seem delusional, the diagnosis of body dysmorphic disorder is still correct. Posttraumatic stress disorder refers to a constellation of symptoms that develop following a traumatic experience. Flashbacks or reliving of the traumatic event may occur; this re-experiencing of the trauma may feel very real—almost to the point of feeling like a hallucination.

The Effects of Drug Use

The use of alcohol or marijuana or other illegal drugs may cause a person to have symptoms that resemble schizophrenia. Psychosis may also occur during or soon after heavy use of a drug (intoxication) or as the person withdraws from the drug after its use. Psychosis that persists more than a month after stopping the drug is suggestive of a primary psychotic disorder, such as schizophrenia, rather than the effects of the drug. The following drugs (particularly when taken in large quantities) can cause psychotic symptoms during their use or immediately after (during withdrawal):

- Alcohol
- Benzodiazepine-type medications (often prescribed for anxiety or insomnia), such as lorazepam (Ativan), clonazepam (Klonopin), or alprazolam (Xanax)
- Stimulant medications, such as methylphenidate (Ritalin) or amphetamine salts (Adderall), used to treat disorders such as attention deficit disorder
- Cocaine (crack) or amphetamines (speed)
- Inhalants
- Heroin
- Narcotic pain killers, such as morphine, hydrocodone, or codeine
- Marijuana
- Hallucinogens such as phencyclidine (or angel dust), ecstasy, and ketamine, which can cause altered perception (such as visual hallucinations) and disordered thoughts that may resemble schizophrenia
- Hallucinogens such as lysergic acid diethylamide (LSD, or acid) and psilocybin (in mushrooms), which can cause unusual sensory experiences, altered sense of self, and intense emotions

- Steroid drugs, such as prednisone and methylprednisolone, used in treating asthma and other medical disorders

In people diagnosed with schizophrenia, these substances can worsen their symptoms and should therefore be completely avoided.

Marijuana use among adolescents and young adults seems to increase the chance of later developing schizophrenia. It is unclear whether marijuana somehow triggers schizophrenia in a susceptible individual or whether people who are prone to developing schizophrenia are more likely to smoke marijuana. Some people with schizophrenia who smoke marijuana have fewer negative symptoms, so the drug use may be a way of "self-medicating." Yet these same people often have more positive symptoms and more frequent hospitalizations compared with those who do not smoke marijuana. Note that drug use does not cause schizophrenia. Rather, the use of these substances may speed up the onset of schizophrenia symptoms in someone who was already at higher risk for the disorder.

Medical Conditions

Certain medical conditions, traumatic brain injury, mental retardation, and dementia may also be associated with psychotic symptoms. Older people suffering from dementia—including Alzheimer's disease, the most common cause of dementia, and Parkinson's disease—may also experience psychosis. Both disorders tend to affect people in the later years of life (age 60 and beyond). The primary symptoms of Alzheimer's disease are impaired short-term memory and disorientation. People who have Parkinson's disease frequently have slow movements, stiff limbs, and tremor. They often experience visual hallucinations.

Delirium is a confusional state that may be associated with psychosis. Someone who has delirium rapidly (over hours or days) develops confusion and disorientation and may appear sleepy at times. An underlying cause, such as an infection or other medical illness, usually explains the confused state. Once the underlying medical problem is addressed, the confusion-associated psychosis usually resolves. Other medical conditions that may be associated with psychotic symptoms include seizures, thyroid disorders, brain tumors, and neurological diseases.

The Course of Schizophrenia

The symptoms of schizophrenia usually become evident in an affected person between the teen years and the late twenties. A small number of people develop it after age 40. It affects all classes, sexes, and nationalities. The course of illness varies, though a decline in functioning is common for many people. Symptoms tend to flare up in an episodic pattern, though the course can vary widely among individuals.

Persons with schizophrenia vary greatly in the degree of functional impairment. With treatment, some return to close to normal functioning while others may only partially regain their earlier level of functioning. A smaller number may become so severely ill that they can no longer live independently. It is difficult to predict the course in your family member. Those who have better insight and have learned how to manage their illness tend to do better over time. Many affected individuals can lead productive lives even without being completely free of symptoms.

Important Points
- Delusions, hallucinations, disordered thinking and behavior, and negative symptoms are the core symptoms of schizophrenia. Changes in behavior, mood, and concentration are also frequently observed. Symptoms are highly variable, and no two people's symptoms are exactly alike.

- Using specific criteria, the diagnosis of schizophrenia is based on an interview of the individual by a psychiatrist, a medical doctor specialized in diagnosing and treating people who have mental illness. No specific blood tests or x-rays help make the diagnosis. With a proper evaluation, however, the diagnosis generally becomes clear, though it may take time and multiple visits with a psychiatrist to confirm the diagnosis.
- Several other psychiatric and medical disorders have symptoms that may resemble schizophrenia and therefore must be differentiated from it in order to confirm the diagnosis.

RESOURCES

American Psychiatric Association. *Diagnostic and Statistical Manual of Mental Disorders.* 5th ed. Text Revision. Arlington, VA: American Psychiatric Publishing, 2022.

Chase, R. *Schizophrenia: A Brother Finds Answers in Biological Science.* Baltimore, MD: Johns Hopkins University Press, 2013. A scientist explores the causes of schizophrenia in order to understand his brother's illness.

Nasar, S. *A Beautiful Mind: The Life of Mathematical Genius and Nobel Laureate John Nash.* New York: Simon and Schuster, 1998. This biography recounts the life of Nobel laureate John Nash, who suffered from schizophrenia.

National Institute of Mental Health. "Schizophrenia." Last revised February 2016. www.nimh.nih.gov/health/topics/schizophrenia/index.shtml.

Saks, Elyn R. *The Center Cannot Hold.* New York: Hachette Books, 2007. Law school professor Elyn Saks recounts her experience living with schizophrenia.

WebMD. "Schizophrenia Health Center." August 18, 2015. www.webmd.com/schizophrenia/guide/schizophrenia-tests. Patient-focused website containing basic information about schizophrenia.

2

What Causes Schizophrenia?

No one knows what causes schizophrenia. Most experts believe it may be due to external and internal factors interacting in multiple complex ways. Thus, if environmental stresses are encountered during a critical period of fetal development (such as fetal distress), and the person also has a sufficient level of genetic risk (such as a family history of the illness), the person is more likely to experience symptoms consistent with schizophrenia. In someone with fewer risk genes, more environmental stress appears to be necessary to develop these symptoms; in someone with a greater number of risk genes, less environmental stress is necessary to develop these symptoms.

Important external factors that may put a person at higher risk include:

- *Perinatal stressors*: "Perinatal" refers to the time period several months before and one month after birth. Examples of such stressors include low fetal oxygen levels, maternal infection, and obstetric complications, all of which are known to interfere with normal brain development.[1]

- *Nutritional deficiencies*, such as maternal iron deficiency: In general, adequate maternal nutrition is essential for normal brain development in the fetus and infant.
- *Urban setting*: Being raised in an urban rather than a rural setting can double your risk.
- *Winter or spring birth*: Being born in winter or early spring increases your risk by 5 to 15 percent.
- *Life stresses*: For example, a personal or family history of migration can increase your risk.
- *Cultural influences*: These include how challenging a person's social context is (such as family or societal expectations) and how much importance this social context places on problems such as the thinking difficulties associated with schizophrenia.
- *Substance abuse*: The use of marijuana, for example, may increase the risk of developing symptoms, bring about an earlier onset of illness than might have otherwise been experienced, or bring about a more severe form of the illness.[2]

The good news is that since environment clearly plays a significant role, existing and future treatment interventions that alter its influence can potentially reduce a person's chances of developing schizophrenia and may even override genetically related risks.

Important internal factors that are thought to increase risk include:

- *Variations in genetic makeup*: Genes are the basic physical and functional units of heredity; half of our genes come from our mother, and half of our genes come from our father.
- *Being male*: Men are more likely to develop schizophrenia, which also tends to occur earlier (by two to three years) in men than in women.

- *Abnormal brain structures*: Schizophrenia is more likely to develop in people with larger than normal ventricle spaces (which are a system of cavities within the brain that connect with the spinal cord canal and contain the cerebralspinal fluid); subtle decreases in total brain volume and gray matter; and changes in white matter. Gray matter is the brain's cells and axons, which are nerve fibers that carry signals between those cells. White matter is the longer-range axons that transmit signals to the gray matter. White matter axons are *myelinated*, meaning they are coated in myelin, a whitish protective insulation that improves the transmission of brain cell signals. Gray matter axons are *unmyelinated*.
- *Abnormal brain functioning*: Disruptions in *thought* are related to activity in the brain's frontal lobe. Difficulties with *emotions*, such as correctly interpreting others' emotions, are related to brain structures such as the amygdala and hippocampus. Problems with *perceptions* (such as hallucinations, delusions) are related to frontal-temporal (front and side) areas of the brain.
- *Abnormal response to outside stressors*: Normal cell activity in the body generates *free radicals,* which are atoms that can react with cells, causing damage. When not properly disposed of by brain cells, these free radicals can damage them, diminishing your ability to function adequately.
- *Abnormal neurochemical activity*: Schizophrenia is more likely in people who have problems with *neurotransmitters* (NTs), which are chemicals that facilitate communication between cells. These include dopamine, which plays a central role in modulating movement, mood, and thinking; glutamate, the primary excitatory NT, which increases brain activity; and gamma-aminobutyric acid, the primary inhibitory NT, which decreases brain activity.[3] Dopamine is a critical NT in terms

of its contribution to this illness and how medications benefit those who have schizophrenia.

The following examples show how external and internal factors may interact in ways that predispose a person to experience symptoms of schizophrenia:

- *Heightened immune system activity,* which may occur in response to infections early in life.
- *Abnormal response to psychological or physical stress,* mediated through the *hypothalamic-pituitary-adrenal axis.* This is a group of brain structures and glands that make up the endocrine system (the system that regulates our hormones) and control the body's physical reactions to stress. In response to stress, the adrenal gland releases an elevated level of the hormone cortisol.
- *Epigenetic effects,* which may be an important mechanism for mediating prenatal environmental stresses (such as exposure to infection, maternal alcohol use, and nutritional deficiencies). Epigenetics is a process that controls gene expression—how the genes you inherit actually function in your body, such as whether a particular gene gets "turned on" or "off"—and, as a result, can regulate important neurobiological and cognitive functions. Thus, this process may alter gene activity in such a way that it increases or decreases the risk of developing an illness such as schizophrenia. Epigenetics is important in treating schizophrenia.

Important Points
- Both biological predisposition (e.g., genes) and environmental factors (e.g., stress) contribute to the risk of developing schizophrenia.
- Their contributions to this process vary depending on multiple factors, such as the number, timing, and severity of stresses a person encounters.

- These factors can be exploited for therapeutic purposes to lower the risk of developing schizophrenia or to more effectively treat symptoms when they occur.

Genetics and Schizophrenia

Of all the potential risks associated with developing schizophrenia, genetics plays a central role.[4] One aspect of this is the existence of *endophenotypes*, which are genetically determined biological markers indicating a greater risk to develop schizophrenia. These markers can be measured in various ways. Examples include altered molecular activity (such as abnormal neurotransmitter-related activity); abnormal cognitive function (such as impaired attention, language, and memory); brain changes seen on neuroimaging (such as decreases in gray matter); and altered electrophysiological activity (such as abnormal eye movements). Further, these markers may represent traits that run in families with some members developing schizophrenia while others do not. They may also help improve diagnosis; predict an individual's course of illness; and, most important, improve a person's prognosis, since endophenotypes are also novel targets for treatment.[5] Currently, however, none of the measures described in this section is used in standard clinical practice.

The two broad approaches for studying the role of genetics in schizophrenia are epidemiological and molecular.

Epidemiological Genetics

The epidemiological approach involves family, twin, and adoption studies. *Family studies* consider the risk of developing schizophrenia for first-degree biological relatives (immediate family members such as a parent or sibling) of a person who has this illness compared with the risk in families without any member who suffers from schizophrenia. The results of these studies indicate that having an immediate family member with the illness can increase a person's risk as high as tenfold (that is, about a 10 percent risk versus 1 percent in the general population).[6] *Twin studies* compare identical to fraternal (nonidentical) pairs in terms of illness risk when one twin has schizophrenia. Although the risk is greater for identical (48 percent) compared with fraternal (17 percent) twin pairs, about half of the time, one identical twin will have schizophrenia, but the other will not. This supports the importance of environmental influences such as stress. *Adoption studies* further highlight the role of a person's genes. Here, the risk is compared between biological and adoptive parents for individuals with schizophrenia. In general, the risk "travels with" the biological and not the adoptive relationship regardless of who raises the person with this illness. That is, the risk remains high for people born to a parent with schizophrenia even if they are raised by adoptive parents who do not have schizophrenia.

Molecular Genetics

Molecular genetics considers how genes express themselves physically by studying the DNA sequences of chromosomes within the genes. *Linkage studies* search for an altered genetic marker that is inherited with the illness within a multigenerational family. *Association studies* look for a DNA sequence variation that occurs more frequently in individuals with schizophrenia than in those without the illness. A recent advance, *candidate gene association studies* (that is, genes previously thought to be associated with schizophrenia), uses family rather than general population samples. This approach focuses on families with several members who have schizophrenia, potentially increasing the presence of any transmitted genetic risk factor(s), while also reducing potentially extraneous factors (such as race, ethnicity, culture) more likely to be present in the general population.

More recently, *genome-wide association studies* (GWAS) are possible because of advances in technology. This approach allows for thousands of potential genetic variations to be analyzed at one time. Thus far, the results of GWAS support the notion that multiple genes (each representing a limited amount of risk) contribute to developing schizophrenia. For example, one study found 108 locations (or loci) on chromosomes associated with an increased risk of schizophrenia.[7] Further, this study found that genes at some of these sites can alter the dopamine 2 receptor and modulate glutamate neurotransmission. Neurotransmission is how neurochemicals, such as glutamate, facilitate communication between brain cells. Such effects have potential treatment-related importance. The researchers also found enriched associations with genes in tissues that are important in the immune response, supporting the possible link between schizophrenia and the immune system. This system comprises many biological structures and processes that protect against various diseases (such as those caused by infectious agents). In this context, a recent important finding identified C4 gene variants (or alleles), which encode for a protein that may increase the risk of schizophrenia by altering synaptic pruning, a critical process during brain development.[8] Further, this process is closely associated with the major histocompatibility complex, a locus which contains multiple genes that affect the immune system.

These findings support the notion that no single gene by itself causes schizophrenia. Further, GWAS *cross-disorder* analyses indicate a substantial overlap in genetic variations among five major psychiatric disorders: schizophrenia, bipolar disorder, attention deficit hyperactivity disorder, autism spectrum disorders, and major depression.[9] This overlap may reflect the known similarity in symptoms of these different disorders but also a shared cause. An important implication of such findings is that our present way of diagnosing schizophrenia may dramatically shift from a reliance on various clinical symptoms to the use of biological markers associated with gene variations. These findings recently led to a worldwide cooperative effort called the Psychiatric Genomic Consortium. This initiative allows for the pooling of genomic data from various sources, which increases sample sizes to better detect a gene's contribution to illness risk.

Another important consideration is that two-thirds of individuals with schizophrenia have no history of this disorder in a close family member. These patients are considered *sporadic* cases, whose illness is possibly caused by *de novo* (spontaneous, not inherited) rare genetic variations, such as the deletion or duplication of small DNA sequences on chromosomes. These variations are called *copy number variations*. They tend to cluster around genes thought to be relevant to brain development. One example is a deletion at the 22q11 chromosome site that predisposes a person to both velocardiofacial (DiGeorge) syndrome and an increased risk for schizophrenia, as well as other neuropsychiatric disorders.[10] Another important implication is that what we presently call schizophrenia may actually be a group of related disorders that, when more clearly distinguished, may benefit from different, more specific treatments.

In this context, a related question is whether genetic testing would be valuable in routine clinical settings to help predict the risk of developing schizophrenia. Although most experts would agree that such testing is premature at this time, these services are already available on the Internet, raising important ethical issues. Currently, genetic testing is not part of the standard treatment of schizophrenia.

Pharmacogenetics and Pharmacogenomics in Treating Schizophrenia

An offshoot of genetic studies is research into pharmacogenetics and pharmacogenomics. These approaches consider how inheritance and acquired genetic variations may alter a medication's effectiveness.[11] *Pharmacogenetics* focuses on a single candidate gene associated with a drug's action and tests for any relationship with treatment response (good or bad). *Pharmacogenomics* uses a multiple gene approach to help identify "profiles" involving several genes with the purpose of better predicting a drug's clinical benefit or side effects. This area of inquiry may lead to various benefits:

- Improved understanding of a drug's *mechanism of action* (how exactly it works) and facilitated development of new, more effective drug therapies
- Prediction of the best drug for an individual, as well as its optimal dose and duration of treatment
- Enhanced medication *adherence* (a person's ability to take a medication as directed) and reduced relapse rates

Although this science is still in the early phases of development, it holds the promise of more "personalized" choices in treatments to increase the benefit and reduce the side effects of medication. In the future, your doctor may be able to prescribe the specific medication you are most likely to respond to and tolerate better. This would be different from the current approach of trying multiple medications until finding the one that works best for the person and that can be tolerated.

Important Points

- Genetic makeup plays a critical role in determining if a person will develop schizophrenia.
- Having an immediate family member, such as a parent or sibling, with schizophrenia increases the chance of developing schizophrenia tenfold.
- On a genetic level, schizophrenia is most likely caused by the interplay of multiple genes rather than one single gene.

- In the future, genetic variations may also serve as markers for the illness, improve diagnosis, and help predict response to specific treatments.

Neuroimaging and Schizophrenia

A major drawback in studying schizophrenia is the uncertainty of a diagnosis based only on clinical symptoms. Advances in neuroimaging technology are providing important information about abnormalities in brain structure and function associated with this condition. Some goals of neuroimaging are to use these findings as biological markers to more precisely identify individuals with this disorder (such as those at high risk); to better predict the course of illness (the prognosis); and to allow better monitoring of treatment effects. Recent advances in how imaging data is collected and analyzed from the various types of available brain scans allow for a more comprehensive evaluation of differences between people who have schizophrenia and those who do not.

Several approaches are now available to image the brain. The neuroimaging technology that is used will depend on what is being examined:

- To look at various *structural changes* in the brain, such as differences in cell volumes
  - Computerized tomography (CT)
  - Structural magnetic resonance imaging (MRI)
- To consider altered *brain activity*
  - Positron emission tomography (PET)
  - Functional magnetic resonance imaging (fMRI)
- To consider *white matter tracts,* which connect different regions of the brain
  - Diffusion-weighted tension imaging (DTI)

- To measure the *activity of various neurochemicals* thought to be relevant to schizophrenia
  - Magnetic resonance spectroscopy (MRS)

Results from thousands of studies conducted using such imaging technologies indicate that schizophrenia is characterized by abnormal connections among important brain networks.[12] The primary outcome from *structural studies* of schizophrenia is the finding that individuals with this disorder have subtle but widespread differences from the brains of those without schizophrenia. These include enlargement of ventricle spaces; loss of gray matter volume, primarily in the medial temporal (middle side) and frontal brain areas; as well as decreases in the gray matter volume of other relevant brain structures (such as the limbic system, thalamus, and striatum). The decrease in brain volume appears to be associated with a reduction in brain cell size rather than number. The end result is abnormal communication (connectivity) between cells.

With more recent advances in technology, the ability to measure activity in these various brain areas is now possible. These studies observed abnormal task-induced activities associated with structural changes in the same brain areas. For example, the frontal areas of the brain are responsible for working memory (that is, the ability of the brain to keep a limited amount of information available long enough to use it), and the temporal areas are responsible for recall of previously learned tasks. Both areas show differences in activity (usually decreased but sometimes increased) in persons with schizophrenia versus those without. Similar patterns of disrupted white matter tract integrity were also observed in these same brain areas.

These findings indicate that the various symptoms (such as hallucinations, delusions, disorganized thoughts) cannot be attributed solely to abnormalities in specific locations of the brain. Rather, they are the outcome of disruptions in complex, large-scale *brain networks*, which are interconnected and can separate and integrate their activities as needed to function effectively. These disruptions appear to primarily affect the connectivity between frontal and temporal areas of the brain. The individual networks include a set of *brain systems*, which together form the basis for specific behaviors, such as attention and memory. A brain system is a distinct brain area (a group of brain cells) and its connections (white matter) to other brain areas, each of which is responsible for a different set of functions.

One important goal in brain imaging research is to "map" the genetic vulnerabilities previously discussed onto these structural and functional findings to better understand the pathological changes in schizophrenia. At this time, most imaging studies are summations of findings from groups of patients. Thus, how to translate this to a better understanding of the symptoms and signs of schizophrenia is a critical next step in developing this approach to diagnose and treat the disorder.

Important Points

- Imaging of individuals with or without schizophrenia can reveal differences in various brain structures and their connections.
- The related functions of these brain areas also differ between those with and those without this illness.

Conclusion

Schizophrenia is a disorder associated with abnormal development of and progressive changes over time in brain structures and activity that disrupt effective communication between relevant groupings of brain cells called brain networks. These brain cells interact with each other through neurochemical (such as dopamine, serotonin, glutamate) signals. Environmental stressors along with genetic deficits in proper cell development, alignment, and communications in the brain occur early in life and lay the groundwork for the characteristic symptoms of schizophrenia, which usually become evident in adolescence or young adulthood.

3

Biological Therapies
for Schizophrenia

The overall help you might expect from any medical treatment includes its potential *benefit* for a specific illness; its *risks*, which must be balanced against any benefit; and your willingness to accept the medication and take it as prescribed. We consider these issues in the context of how you can best manage the various symptoms of schizophrenia that you may be experiencing. This chapter speaks directly to you, the individual affected by schizophrenia. Family members will undoubtedly find this information useful, however, as they support their loved one in the healing process.

Stages of Schizophrenia

As with many other medical conditions, schizophrenia is treated in different ways depending on the stage of the illness. Thus, different educational, social, psychotherapeutic, and biological approaches are considered depending on *when* in the course of your illness they are to be provided. For our discussion of these various treatment approaches, we consider the following stages of schizophrenia:

Early Course of the Illness

- *High-risk, prodromal (precursory) period*: A variable period, ranging from months to years, during which you experience early, mild symptoms of the illness
- *First episode*: The first time you experience full symptoms of the illness
- *Early onset period:* The five years following your first episode

Later Course of the Illness

- *Acute management* of periodic worsening in your symptoms
- *Long-term management* to reduce the risk of recurring episodes, improve your ability to function, and help you achieve important life goals
- *Treatment resistance,* a common problem we discuss below, including strategies to help you to overcome it

Although certain approaches are more appropriate depending on the stage of illness, to achieve the most benefit, you will usually need to receive two or more of them (such as medication plus education about this illness for you and your family). In this chapter we focus on biological treatments, including their potential benefits, their risks, and issues affecting your comfort in taking them. In chapter 4 we focus on educational, social, and psychotherapeutic treatments in more detail.

Early Course of the Illness

Increasingly, the focus of treating schizophrenia is to identify as early as possible if you are at higher risk for developing this illness. The aim is to intervene before it progresses too far, thus avoiding or reducing any disability that may occur because of the disorder. One difficulty with this approach is in accurately predicting whether you will actually go on to develop the full symptoms of schizophrenia. Much progress has been made in developing predictors for schizophrenia over the past twenty years, with several investigators developing criteria to determine who may be at greater risk. For example, according to one group of researchers, to qualify as *ultra-high risk*, you should experience at least one of the following:

- Mild, less clear symptoms
- Brief, limited, intermittent periods of clear psychotic symptoms
- A greater genetic risk (such as a strong family history of the illness)
- A decrease in your ability to socialize with family and friends[1]

Other potential predictors of whether you may be at higher risk for experiencing psychosis include:

- High levels of unusual thought content (such as feeling that you can read others' thoughts or that they can read yours)
- High levels of suspicion or paranoia
- History of substance use (such as marijuana)[2]

Psychological approaches and certain medications may decrease your chances of experiencing a full episode of schizophrenia.[3] For example, one study found that combining an intensive community care program, family education, and omega-3 polyunsaturated fatty acid supplements could decrease your chances of having a psychotic episode during a one-year period.[4] At these early stages, antipsychotic drugs are generally avoided because of their potential for serious side effects. If you do not benefit from these other interventions, however, there is some evidence that low doses of a single drug, such as risperidone, combined with cognitive behavioral therapy (CBT) may lessen your chances of having a full psychotic episode.[5] With CBT, you are guided by a trained therapist through a series of steps that consider alternate interpretations or explanations for the symptoms you are experiencing. The hope is that through this process, your understanding of these symptoms will change enough so that they are less likely to interfere with your day-to-day interactions and routine activities.

Unfortunately, you may go on to experience a first full episode of symptoms, which are often not accurately recognized as schizophrenia for months to years. This lack of accurate diagnosis can delay your treatment and ultimately worsen the long-term course.[6] Thus, mental health care providers need to work on their ability to more quickly recognize this problem and to introduce effective plans, such as the use of medication plus social and educational interventions. Several studies support the effectiveness of early recognition and timely treatment interventions to minimize cognitive impairment, suicidal behaviors, and the length of hospital stays, as well as to increase the chances of making a better recovery, finding employment, and continuing to function more effectively for up to ten years after the onset of the illness.[7]

To emphasize, the first few years following a full episode of symptoms are critical in terms of providing an effective treatment plan for you. Even at this early point in the illness, you may be experiencing difficulties in the ability to think clearly. Thus, if an effective working alliance with your care providers is not firmly established, your willingness to accept treatment recommendations is often compromised by your symptoms, increasing the risk for further psychotic episodes. This could create a downward cycle, possibly leading to further deterioration in your ability to function and an increased risk of thoughts about harming yourself. To prevent such an outcome, the appropriate use of medication combined with educational and psychological approaches for you and your family, as well as community support programs, are critical for stabilizing your illness.

Important Points

- Accurate, early identification of your illness and timely appropriate interventions are crucial, since delaying them may worsen your long-term course.
- Your treatment team should also help with any related problems you may experience, such as depression, substance use, and difficulties following through with recommended treatments.
- When prescribed as part of a comprehensive treatment plan, appropriate doses of an antipsychotic with a favorable side effect profile can be helpful. These medications and their side effects are described in more detail later in this chapter.

Later Course of the Illness

If your illness progresses beyond the earlier stages, you may experience intermittent worsening of symptoms, such as flare-ups of paranoia and auditory hallucinations. These episodes may require emergency room visits and even short hospital stays. Once these symptoms improve, your treatment should then focus on preventing further episodes. When this is accomplished, you and your treatment team can then focus on improving your ability to function more effectively in various areas of life. As with other medical disorders, an important reason for treating schizophrenia is to help better manage this illness so that you can achieve important life goals, such as furthering your education, achieving stable work, experiencing more rewarding relationships with your family and friends, or getting married.

Acute Management

A mainstay of your treatment plan at this stage is the judicious use of antipsychotic medication. Since the benefit of the available drugs for schizophrenia is generally similar (with the exception

Table 3.1 First-Generation Antipsychotics

Common trade name	Generic name	Usual daily dosing range	Comments
Thorazine	Chlorpromazine	100–1,000 mg	First antipsychotic to be approved worldwide
Mellaril	Thioridazine	30–800 mg	Higher risk of cardiac rhythm problems
Serentil	Mesoridazine	20–200 mg	Higher risk of cardiac rhythm problems
Stelazine	Trifluoperazine	2–60 mg	
Prolixin	Fluphenazine	5–40 mg	Available in LAI formulation
Trilafon	Perphenazine	2–60 mg	
Navane	Thiothixene	6–60 mg	
Loxitane, Adasuve	Loxapine	20–250 mg 10 mg	Also available as an acute, single-dose inhalant formulation
Moban	Molindone	15–225 mg	May cause fewer problems with weight gain
Haldol	Haloperidol	3–50 mg	Most commonly used FGA; available in LAI formulation

Note: FGA = first-generation antipsychotic; LAI = long-acting injectable

of clozapine), the choice of a specific antipsychotic is often based on the potential for causing side effects, which can differ substantially among these agents.[8] As discussed in chapter 2, however, advances in pharmacogenetics and pharmacogenomics will ultimately improve identification of candidate genes, which then can be used to better predict which medication will be most beneficial while posing the fewest risks for you. Twenty-nine antipsychotic medications (divided into first-generation and second-generation groups) are presently available in the United States. Tables 3.1 and 3.2 list the most frequently used, including their common trade and generic names, as well as the usual daily dosing recommendations.

Table 3.2 Second-Generation Antipsychotics

Common trade name	Generic name	Usual daily dosing range	Comments
Clozaril	Clozapine	100–900 mg	Most effective AP for treatment-refractory patients
Risperdal	Risperidone	2–8 mg	Available in LAI formulation
Zyprexa	Olanzapine	5–20 mg	Available in LAI formulation
Seroquel	Quetiapine	75–800 mg	
Geodon	Ziprasidone	40–160 mg	Fewer problems with weight gain
Abilify	Aripiprazole	5–30 mg	Available in LAI formulations
Invega	Paliperidone	3–12 mg	Available in LAI formulations, including one that only requires an injection every 3 months
Fanapt	Iloperidone	12–24 mg	
Saphris	Asenapine	10–20 mg	Only available in a sublingual formulation
Latuda	Lurasidone	40–160 mg	Fewer problems with weight gain
Rexulti	Brexpiprazole	2–4 mg	Akathisia most common adverse effect in trials
Vraylar	Cariprazine	1.5–6 mg	Akathisia most common adverse effect in trials
Caplyta	Lumateperone	42 mg	Sedation common in trials

Note: AP = antipsychotic; LAI = long-acting injectable

As noted above, the one exception to the similar efficacy among antipsychotics is clozapine. This drug demonstrates enhanced benefit compared with other agents in numerous studies, primarily for those experiencing treatment resistance, but may also help in the early course of the illness.[9] Because of its potentially serious side effects, however, clozapine is usually not recommended as an initial treatment option. Table 3.3 lists the potential benefits and risks of clozapine.

When you experience an acute worsening of symptoms, it is often accompanied by feelings of anxiety, agitation, and other experiences that may frighten you (such as suicidal thoughts) or frighten others (such as aggressive behaviors). At times, these emotions and behaviors can be successfully managed with de-escalation tech-

Table 3.3 Clozapine

Potential benefits	Potential risks
• May improve: 　◦ treatment-refractory patients 　◦ suicidal, aggressive, or violent behaviors 　◦ life expectancy • Diminishes motor side effects • Lowers risk for or improves tardive dyskinesia • Minimizes risk of elevated prolactin levels	Box warnings: • Agranulocytosis (low white blood cell count) • Seizures • Myocarditis (inflammation of the heart muscle) • Orthostasis (lowered blood pressure) • Increased mortality when used in dementia patients Other potentially serious adverse effects: • Weight gain / metabolic syndrome • Ketoacidosis (a severe adverse effect associated with diabetes) • Gastrointestinal tract slowing (which may cause severe constipation or even blockage of the bowel)

niques, such as placing you in a room with minimal stimulation and having people present with whom you are comfortable and who can reassure you that these feelings will subside. Medications may also be necessary to ensure your safety and the safety of others. They can be given by mouth, by injection, or, with a recent innovation, by acute inhalation through the mouth (much like an asthma inhaler).[10] Additional medications that might help include antianxiety agents if you are agitated, sedatives to help you sleep better, and antidepressants to improve your mood. In addition, you may receive other medications to relieve side effects associated with the antipsychotic drug. A common example is the use of an anticholinergic medication (such as benztropine or Cogentin) to relieve the side effect of muscle stiffness.

Once these symptoms are better, you, your family, and members of supporting community programs will need to work together to establish an effective treatment plan while you are recovering (usually the first six months following an acute episode). During this phase, in addition to taking an antipsychotic medication, you will also benefit from ongoing educational efforts to help all involved parties better understand the nature of this illness and its effect on your ability to function. Once you achieve short-term control of your symptoms, the focus can then turn to their long-term management.

Long-Term Management

As with many medical conditions (such as diabetes, high blood pressure, low thyroid activity), the symptoms of schizophrenia can persist throughout your life. Thus, the focus of long-term treatment turns to controlling these symptoms to avoid future episodes. This allows you to achieve more sustained periods of functioning. A successful course of treatment will move from *response* (helping you stay healthy enough to avoid the hospital and remain in the community); to *remission* (minimizing or eliminating your active symptoms); to *recovery* (improving your ability to function better and experience more satisfaction from various life activities). This progression can dramatically improve your quality of life and provide the opportunity to achieve important personal goals. While antipsychotic medications remain an indispensable component of the treatment plan during this phase, social and psychological approaches assume increasing importance in helping you to realize these goals (see chapter 4).

During this process, you may find that taking medication by mouth every day is not practical over prolonged periods (such as years). Several of these agents are available in long-acting injectable (LAI) formulations, which may improve your chances for adequate treatment (see tables 3.1 and 3.2). These injections are usually given every two to four weeks; however, one recently approved formulation of paliperidone allows for injections once every three months. These LAI agents may allow for more adequate blood levels of the drug than you could achieve when taking the medication by mouth. This is because of differences in how you absorb the oral drug formulation in your gastrointestinal tract and break it down in your liver. Further, since regular clinic visits are required to receive the injections, it becomes immediately clear when you stop your medication. Another advantage is that if you stop taking the injections, the medication will remain in your body at adequate levels for longer periods (weeks to months) than if taken by mouth. This allows the treatment team an opportunity to explore and address with you the reasons for stopping the medication, possibly leading to resumption before you experience a recurrence of symptoms.

Treatment Resistance

Even with adequate medication treatment (a sufficient dose for a sufficient period of time), you may not experience enough benefit or may not be able to tolerate an adequate trial. Many efforts are ongoing to improve the benefit of such drug treatments and to reduce problems with their associated side effects. These efforts can be divided into three approaches:

1. Modifying existing medications to improve their benefit
2. Developing new medication and nonmedication biological strategies with different mechanisms of action from standard antipsychotics
3. Repurposing other available medications for use as alternatives or supplements to standard antipsychotics

Modifying Existing Medications

One of the more common strategies is to develop alternate formulations of an antipsychotic to improve ease of use and/or to reduce side effects. Some examples include:

- *Acute injectable or inhalational formulations* for more effective management of periods of agitation

- *Long-acting injectable formulations* for problems you may have with taking the medication by mouth
- *Active metabolites* (such as paliperidone), which may decrease certain side effects of the parent drug (in this case, the drug risperidone)
- *Sustained oral formulations* (such as quetiapine XR) to decrease the frequency of dosing, potentially improving your ability to remain on treatment

Biological Therapies with Different Mechanisms of Action

Although the dopamine neurotransmitter system was a major focus in developing existing antipsychotic medications, it is clear that drugs working only through the dopamine system are not sufficient to control all symptoms of schizophrenia. Medications that work through different neurotransmitter systems are being studied as alternatives to standard antipsychotics or as strategies to enhance their benefit. Some of the most active areas of study involve:

- *Serotonin*: A neurotransmitter closely associated with the dopamine system and able to modulate its activities to enhance benefit and/or decrease side effects
- *Glutamate*: The primary excitatory neurotransmitter in the brain, thought to be partly responsible for various symptoms seen in schizophrenia
- *Gamma-aminobutyric acid*: The primary inhibitory neurotransmitter in the brain, which helps to modulate the activity of several related systems (such as dopamine and glutamate)
- *Acetylcholine*: A neurotransmitter that affects various aspects of cognitive function that are often disrupted in those with schizophrenia
- *Norepinephrine*: A neurotransmitter that can facilitate alertness, improve mood, and enhance certain cognitive activities

- *Histamine*: A neurotransmitter that regulates other key neurotransmitter systems and whose modulation with certain medications has shown preliminary benefit for symptoms of schizophrenia

Many patients who suffer from schizophrenia do not adequately benefit from or cannot tolerate presently available medications. As a result, therapeutic neuromodulation is being studied as an adjunctive (secondary) therapy for persistent auditory hallucinations and persistent negative symptoms. This approach involves altering the electrical activity of the brain for therapeutic purposes. For example, electroconvulsive therapy (ECT) is an effective treatment for patients requiring rapid resolution of their symptoms, usually to ensure their safety. Other potential nonmedication biological therapies not presently approved by the FDA for treatment of schizophrenia have promising initial study results:

- *Transcranial magnetic stimulation* (TMS) uses magnetic pulses to induce or inhibit electrical currents in the brain, thereby reducing symptoms of schizophrenia.
- *Transcranial direct cortical stimulation* (tDCS) applies a sustained, weak current flow through areas of the brain thought to play a role in the symptoms of schizophrenia.
- *Deep brain stimulation* (DBS) involves electrical stimulation by electrodes implanted in brain neurocircuits that are considered to play a role in the symptoms of schizophrenia.[11]

Repurposing Available Medications

Examples of this repurposing approach for other conditions include certain available hormone therapies (such as estrogen, oxytocin), steroids (such as glucocorticoids, neurosteroids), and nutraceuticals (such as omega-3 fatty acids, folate, vitamin D). In schizophrenia, inflammation and oxidative stress (such as excessive free radical production) may be important mechanisms in the development of various symptoms. In this context, nonsteroidal anti-inflammatory drugs (NSAIDs), such as aspirin or celecoxib, and omega-3 fatty acids or antioxidant supplementation may prove helpful for you when added to standard antipsychotic agents. None of these approaches is presently approved for treatment of schizophrenia, but promising results from preliminary studies may eventually encourage more conclusive studies and lead to the use of these treatments in appropriate individuals.

Important Points

- Antipsychotic and other medications play an important role in rapidly controlling symptoms and protecting you and others from injury during a full episode of psychosis.
- Once your symptoms are controlled for an adequate period, other treatments, such as education and social skills training, become important additions to your overall treatment plan.
- Your ability to continue treatment for sustained periods is necessary to achieve the best results and can be aided by long-acting injectable medication formulations.
- When you are unable to achieve sufficient help from standard treatments, newer approaches may help to further your progress

Risks

Any potential benefit from biological treatments must be carefully weighed against their risks as well. Though all antipsychotics carry some risk for side effects, they are usually mild to moderate in severity, and you will often find that they diminish over a fairly short time. If these symptoms persist, however, you have several options for managing them. You and your treatment team will need to decide whether the benefits are worth the effort. Tables 3.4 and 3.5 list the most common side effects and their rel-

Effect	CPZ	THZ	MSZ	TRI	FLU	PER	THX	LOX	MOL	HPD
Neurological	+	+	+	++	+++	++	+++	++	++	+++
Weight gain	++	++	++	+	+	+	+	+	+	+
Anticholinergic	+++	+++	+++	+	+	+	+	+	+	0
Hematologic	++	0/+	0/+	0/+	0/+	0/+	0/+	0/+	0/+	0
Cardiovascular	++	+++	+++	0/+	0/+	0/+	0/+	0/+	0/+	++
Prolactin	+	+	+	++	+++	++	++	+	+	+++
Sedation	+++	+++	+++	+	+	++	+	+	+	+

Notes: At appropriate doses: 0 = none; + = mild; ++ = moderate; +++ = substantial. CPZ = chlorpromazine;
THZ = thioridazine; MSZ = mesoridazine; TRI = trifluoperazine; FLU = fluphenazine; PER = perphenazine;
THX = thiothixene; LOX = loxapine; MOL = molindone; HPD = haloperidol.

ative severity for the first-generation and second-generation antipsychotic drugs.

Neurological Side Effects

Because antipsychotics affect the dopamine neurotransmitter system, neurological symptoms can occur.[12] You may experience either underactive or overactive movement problems. A common example of an underactive movement side effect is called *pseudoparkinsonism*. As the name implies, you may appear to have the neurological disorder Parkinson's disease. It typically presents with a dulled expression, muscle stiffness, slowed walking, unsteady gait, and tremors of the hands when they are at rest. Fortunately, this side effect is much less frequent with most second-generation antipsychotics. It can be readily reversed by lowering the dose of antipsychotic when possible, adding a medication to counteract this effect (such as an anticholinergic drug), or switching to an alternate agent with less tendency to produce parkinsonian symptoms. A common example of overactive movements is *akathisia*. With this side effect, you experience an inner feeling of tension or restlessness, the need to move your legs or to pace back and forth. Again, adjusting the

Table 3.5 Common Side Effects and Their Relative Severity: Second-Generation Antipsychotics

Effect	CLZ	RIS	OLZ	QTP	ZIP	ARP	PAL	ILO	ASN	LUR	BREX	CAR	LUM
Neurological	0	+	0/+	0	0/+	0/+	+	+	0	+	+	+	0
Weight gain	+++	++	+++	++	0/+	0/+	++	+	+	0/+	+	+	0
Anticholinergic	+++	0/+	+/++	0/+	0/+	0	0/+	0/+	0	0	0	0	0/+
Hematologic	+++	0	0	0	0	0	0	0	0	0	0	0	0
Cardiovascular	0/+	+	+	+	++	0	+	0/+	0	0/+	0/+	0	0
Prolactin	0/+	+++	0/+	0/+	0/+	0	+++	++	0	++	0	0	0
Sedation	+++	+	+/++	++	++	+	+	+	+	+	+	+	++

Notes: At appropriate doses: 0 = none; + = mild; ++ = moderate; +++ = substantial. CLZ = clozapine; RIS = risperidone; OLZ = olanzapine; QTP = quetiapine; ZIP = ziprasidone; ARP = aripiprazole; PAL = paliperidone; ILO = iloperidone; ASN = asenapine; LUR = lurasidone; BREX = brexpiprazole; CAR = cariprazine; LUM = lumateperone.

antipsychotic dose downward when possible, adding a medication to counteract these sensations (such as a benzodiazepine or beta-blocking drug), or switching to another antipsychotic that is less likely to cause these symptoms can relieve these hyperactive movements.

With longer-term exposure (months to years), you may experience *tardive dyskinesia* (TD), which is characterized by abnormal, involuntary movements of the muscles in the face, arms, legs, or rest of your body. Factors that may increase your risk of developing TD include older age, female gender, the presence of a mood disorder diagnosis, and other brain problems (such as dementia or stroke). If recognized early, stopping your antipsychotic when clinically possible or switching to agents with less risk for this problem (such as clozapine or quetiapine) can reverse this process. Adding other agents (VMAT-2 inhibitors, such as valbenazine, or procholinergic agents, such as donepezil) may also help you. In some instances, however, these movements may persist.

Weight and Metabolic Side Effects

If you have schizophrenia, your life expectancy in comparison to the general population may be reduced. This is the result of several factors, including lifestyle choices, such as an unhealthy diet, inadequate physical activity, smoking cigarettes, and the excessive use of various substances (such as alcohol or marijuana). Further complicating your risk is the problem of weight gain, which is a side effect of many the antipsychotic agents. In general, as your weight increases, so does the risk for abnormal metabolic changes (such as elevated cholesterol and triglyceride levels); elevations in blood pressure; and high blood sugar levels. These changes can increase your risk of developing type 2 diabetes, as well as heart- and brain-related problems. Thus, your treatment team needs to inform you about these issues before you begin taking an antipsychotic drug. Further, your team should work with you to minimize these risks by helping you develop a better diet (such as by providing nutritional counseling), increasing your level of physical activity, and making sure you receive appropriate medical follow-up. The goal is to prevent (or at least minimize) weight gain by encouraging you to engage in a healthier lifestyle.

When clinically appropriate, choosing an antipsychotic with less risk for weight gain is the best option. When this is not feasible or when you still gain weight even with a drug less likely to cause this problem, the addition of certain drugs (such as metformin or topiramate) may prevent you from gaining weight or may enhance weight loss.[13]

Cardiac Effects

In addition to the effects on your heart function of excessive weight gain, antipsychotics can cause heart rhythm problems (such as a long QT syndrome), drops in blood pressure, inflammation or damage of the heart muscle (myocarditis or cardiomyopathy), or inflammation of the heart's covering (pericarditis). Fortunately, these events are not common, but when they do occur, they can be quite serious. You can prevent or manage these effects by changing your dose of antipsychotic, monitoring for these potential problems when indicated (such as having electrocardiograms or specific blood tests to look for inflammation or muscle damage of the heart), and changing your antipsychotic if any of these symptoms arise.

Prolactin Effects

By blocking dopamine in certain areas of the brain, many antipsychotics will increase your prolactin hormone levels. This in turn may cause you to experience irregular menstrual periods, a complete stop of your menstrual cycle, or problems with sexual activity. Men may develop enlargement of breast tissue (gynecomastia), and women may have milk discharge from the breasts. Other possible problems you may experience with sustained increases in prolactin levels include abnormalities in bone density (osteoporosis) and an increased risk of certain types of cancer. Switching to or adding a drug with less likelihood of causing this problem (such as aripiprazole) or adding certain drugs (such as estrogen) are possible strategies if you are doing well on the antipsychotic otherwise.

Cholinergic Side Effects

Many antipsychotic agents, as well as other coprescribed drugs, affect the cholinergic neurotransmitter system by blocking some of its receptors. This effect can cause you to experience *peripheral side effects* (such as blurred vision, dryness of the mouth, urinary difficulties, constipation) and *central side effects* (such as delirium and memory problems). Reducing your dose of antipsychotic when possible, switching to an antipsychotic without these effects, and reducing the number of medications you are taking with anticholinergic properties are common strategies to minimize these problems.

Hematologic Side Effects

Antipsychotics can adversely affect the normal activity of various blood cells (such as white cells, red cells, and platelets). One of the more serious examples is the ability of clozapine to lower your white cell count to levels insufficient to protect you from developing an infection (a condition called *agranulocytosis*). Therefore, when taking clozapine, you must have regularly scheduled blood tests to monitor for this complication and to allow for early, appropriate interventions to reverse this process. With such safeguards, the incidence of agranulocytosis associated with clozapine is well below 1 percent. If this condition does occur, however, you may require aggressive medical management (such as hospitalization and medications to stimulate white cell production) to prevent more serious consequences.

Sedative Side Effects

Many antipsychotics produce initial sedating effects. This may actually be helpful to you if you are experiencing agitation, anxiety, and poor sleep as a result of an acute psychotic episode. As you realize the full benefit of the medication over several days, however, persistent sedation can become problematic. Fortunately, the chances are good that you will develop tolerance to this effect—but you may not. Ongoing excessive sedation when engaging in activities that require you to remain alert and to have adequate reaction times (such as driving an automobile) may pose significant problems. Also, if you are constantly feeling sleepy or fatigued, your chances of continuing the medication are substantially reduced. Lowering the dose of the antipsychotic agent or switching to an alternate drug with less of a sedating effect can help you manage this problem.

Other Side Effects

You may experience other potential side effects when taking an antipsychotic agent. Though these effects are fortunately far less common than those we discuss above, some can be serious, such as neuroleptic malignant syndrome, which leads to a hyperautonomic state, meaning symptoms such as dramatic increases in temperature, blood pressure, and heart rate. Other uncommon side effects include seizures and adverse drug interactions, which can alter the levels of the drugs that are coprescribed, thus compromising efficacy or increasing toxicity. Your treatment team can minimize these risks by educating you about the possibility of these problems and how to monitor carefully for their early signs.

Various therapeutic neuromodulation therapies also carry certain risks. For example, ECT can disrupt your recent memories. TMS is generally considered safe but may cause discomfort at the site of stimulation, headaches, and, rarely, a seizure. DBS requires that you undergo a surgical procedure to implant the device and stimulating electrodes. As with any other surgical procedure, there is the potential for related complications (such as infection or bleeding).

Important Points

- Although you will probably experience some side effects with antipsychotic medications, most are not serious, will gradually subside, or can be readily managed.
- Some side effects, however, can be serious and require you to be fully informed about their potential before starting treatment as well as carefully monitored during their use to prevent subsequent complications.

Adherence

Adherence refers to taking your medication as prescribed by your doctor. Although adherence is problematic for people with all kinds of conditions, multiple factors make it potentially more difficult for those with schizophrenia. These factors may include illness-related problems with thinking, such as poor attention, concentration, and memory; a diminished ability to recognize the effects of the illness on your life; a lack of necessary resources (such as adequate finances to obtain medications) that often confronts you; and side effects you may encounter from the various treatments for schizophrenia. As a result of any or all of these circumstances, your ability to adhere to your treatment may vary over time (ranging from adequate to inadequate). Thus, your treatment team needs to establish a working alliance with you and your family to identify the issues that interfere with adequate adherence, and to cooperatively resolve obstacles to improve adherence when possible. Such efforts can minimize your risk of relapsing or having new episodes, both of which may impair your functioning over time. An important component of this process is to help you understand that adequate adherence to medication is important in the process of attaining your personal goals in life (this is discussed further in chapter 5).

Conclusion

Any benefit you realize from biological therapies for your schizophrenia must be carefully balanced against the potential risks to you. Further, the best outcomes rely on your willingness to contribute to the development of and persistence with the treatment plan, including taking medications properly. Depending on the stage of illness, different approaches are required, including educational, social, psychotherapeutic, and biological. You will usually need various combinations of these approaches to achieve the best outcome.

4

Psychosocial and Behavioral Treatments for Schizophrenia

People who have schizophrenia may experience various symptoms that often differ from person to person. Further, these symptoms usually vary over time in terms of their severity, how often they occur, and how long they last. Although antipsychotic drugs are often helpful over the course of this illness, they are usually not adequate to manage all symptoms or to modulate the illness as it affects people's ability to function and their overall quality of life. Thus, an optimal treatment plan must strike a delicate and changing balance between biological and psychological approaches, depending on the stage of illness, current symptoms, and environmental factors.

While chapter 3 focuses on biological treatments, this chapter emphasizes the importance of psychological and behavioral approaches, including educational, social rehabilitative, and psychotherapeutic interventions. Each person's situation is unique, and the goal is to develop an individualized treatment plan that maximizes the use of all available resources to best manage the person's illness.

As in chapter 3, in this chapter we talk directly to the person who has schizophrenia, although we expect that this chapter will be of interest to family members, too.

Educational Interventions

Psychoeducation is the part of treatment in which you and your family receive information about schizophrenia and how it is managed.[1] Your treatment team also helps you develop realistic expectations about the illness and modulate related emotional reactions and distress. The hope is to improve insight into the illness, which will help you cope better and communicate more effectively. Psychoeducation also helps with problem solving and crisis planning.[2]

The specific problems most frequently targeted in psychoeducation are relapse, rehospitalization, and medication use.[3] There is also evidence that psychoeducation for your family early in the course of your illness increases their knowledge and improves their ability to help you. Families who are informed are better able to assess the associated stresses and develop more effective coping strategies, which in turn reduces their sense of burden and their risk for developing physical and psychological problems. Psychoeducation is often provided in a group multiple-family format, which further enhances its usefulness, primarily through peer support.

Psychosocial Rehabilitation

Psychosocial rehabilitation is based on the recovery and stress-vulnerability models.[4] This approach attempts to address the question of whether having schizophrenia, even with some persistent symptoms, keeps you from living a meaningful and productive life.[5] Evidence-based rehabilitation encompasses several approaches, including:

- Social skills training
- Assertive community treatment (ACT)
- Supported employment (SE)
- Cognitive remediation (CR)
- Peer-implemented services

Social Skills Training

Social skills training helps you improve different areas of social functioning. For example, *interpersonal skills training* focuses on one-to-one interactions, ranging from simple conversations to more complicated relationship interactions. This training usually occurs in small groups where role-play and practice are commonly used techniques. *Independent living skills training* involves a professional to help you with activities such as self-care, housekeeping, financial management, and use of public resources. *Illness/wellness/recovery skills training* helps you better manage the illness and engage in healthier activities. *Social cognition training* improves your perception and understanding of social interactions, such as the behaviors, feelings, and intentions of others. In group formats, you learn to more effectively perceive, identify, interpret, and respond to social and emotional cues.[6]

Assertive Community Treatment

The ACT approach involves a team that focuses on a small group of individuals with the aim of helping them meet their physical and mental health needs. This is accomplished by enhancing the group members' coping skills, motivation, and treatment engagement. In addition, ACT educates community members to help ensure they receive adequate services. These programs are widely available in the United States and are especially helpful for those who require such services frequently. One study concluded that ACT was more effective than standard treatment in helping families cope, improving their satisfaction with services, and reducing the cost of care.[7]

Supported Employment

Having a job can increase your independence, improve your ability to socialize, improve your symptoms, and decrease your need to use the hospital. All of these contribute to a better level of functioning and quality of life. Those with schizophrenia often want to work, but most are unemployed, largely because of their symptoms, as well as concerns about losing disability benefits. Thus, an important goal is to help you achieve competitive employment.[8] Supported employment involves quickly finding work for you and then providing follow-along vocational and mental health services. This approach contrasts with earlier models, which involved lengthy prevocational training. Recent evidence indicates that SE consistently helps adults with mental disorders achieve higher rates of competitive employment, need fewer days to get hired at the first competitive job, work more hours and weeks, and receive higher wages.[9]

Cognitive Remediation

The CR approach acknowledges that cognitive problems are a core symptom of schizophrenia. Thus, because of this illness, you will often have difficulties with paying attention, learning, memory, processing speed, and problem solving. When these problems are not addressed, they can interfere with your social functioning, living skills, and ability to hold a job. There are a number of ways to provide CR, all of which primarily aim to improve functioning in the community, as well as cognition.[10]

Cognitive remediation approaches are divided into *cognition-enhancing techniques* and *compensatory techniques*. The first approach helps you to directly address specific cognitive impairments (such as working memory) through specially designed activities and repeated exercises. The second approach helps you "work around" specific impairments by recruiting other cognitive processes that are still functioning normally. Common to most CR approaches is a *drill and practice* model, using repetitive practice and increasingly more difficult cognitive exercises. An important assumption in CR is that your brain remains capable of physical and functional change throughout life (this ability is called *neuroplasticity*).[11] Cognitive remediation exercises are often computerized. In addition, a coaching therapist helps you translate newly acquired cognitive skills into improved functioning in real-world situations.

Studies support the benefit of CR, and notably, more recent findings report alterations in targeted brain systems using techniques such as drill and practice.[12] There is also evidence that combining CR with other rehabilitative approaches (such as skills training and strategy coaching) may further improve outcomes.[13] For example, one recent study found that combining SE with CR more than doubled employment rates (49 percent versus 20 percent) over two years in lower-functioning individuals compared with SE alone.[14]

Peer-Implemented Interventions

Peer-implemented interventions involve mental health systems that use consumer-directed programs, as well as the help of other people who have schizophrenia. This approach attempts to capitalize on the experience of those who have achieved recovery. With this approach, your peers work along with mental health professionals to provide you support, guidance, respect, and insight. The premise is that those with symptoms of schizophrenia can offer a unique and invaluable perspective, different from that of professionals who have not experienced this illness.[15]

Programs are available throughout the United States, including drop-in centers, mutual support groups, peer education, advocacy programs, and multiservice agencies that provide a variety of resources (such as support during a crisis, guidance in finding employment, and help in securing housing). In particular, crisis intervention approaches during acute flare-ups of your illness can reduce your need to enter the hospital.[16]

Important Points

- Your family's involvement can improve treatment planning and implementation, making it more likely that you will receive the best care.
- Various techniques for strengthening social skills can improve your relationships with friends and family.
- Cognitive remediation approaches can improve your overall functioning and help you better integrate into your community.
- Your peers working in collaboration with mental health professionals can often enhance the quality of your care.

Psychotherapeutic Interventions

Two major psychotherapeutic approaches are used to help people with schizophrenia:

- Family therapy (FT)
- Cognitive behavioral therapy (CBT)

Family Therapy

Family therapy recognizes the significant role your family plays in reducing relapse and hospitalizations. Although some relatives with "high expressed emotions" (such as those who are overly critical) may increase your chances of relapse after an initial episode of worsening symptoms, family members who are educated, coached, and guided can play a more positive role.[17] Further, when your family is actively involved, you are more likely to stay in treatment and feel satisfied with the experience.[18] Important aspects of FT include illness education, relapse prevention planning, and training in problem-solving skills. The two most frequently used approaches are *behavioral family therapy* and *multifamily group therapy*, which compare favorably with standard treatment approaches.[19]

Cognitive Behavioral Therapy

Cognitive behavioral therapy (CBT) can help you identify and modify negative thoughts, identify when you misinterpret experiences, and modify thinking patterns that lead you to destructive behaviors and feelings. *CBT for psychosis* (CBTp) helps you identify specific problems or symptoms; develop better cognitive and behavioral approaches to manage them; and challenge beliefs that support ongoing delusional thoughts and distressing beliefs about voices. CBTp starts with a specific formulation of your experience of psychotic symptoms, such as hallucinations or delusions, and then focuses on related thoughts, behaviors, and emotional reactions. The next step helps you develop new coping strategies. This approach will vary depending on the specific problems that emerge during your therapy, but it often includes:

- Developing a model of psychosis
- Reinterpreting the meaning of delusional beliefs and hallucinations
- Devising relapse prevention strategies[20]

Although CBTp is primarily used to reduce persistent positive symptoms (such as delusions and hallucinations), combining it with other rehabilitation approaches (such as social skills training or psychoeducation) can help you manage other problems, such as substance use, suicidality, and negative symptoms.[21] CBTp can help whether you have a chronic history or are earlier in the course of your illness.[22] Studies that assessed persistent benefits over long periods after the initial treatment intervention found especially strong evidence for the value of CBTp.[23]

Adherence therapy is related to CBTp. This approach uses motivational and CBT techniques to modify your beliefs about medications with the goal of improving your ability to take medication as prescribed.[24] Yet another form of cognitive behavioral therapy is *recovery-oriented cognitive therapy*. Here, you learn to more effectively address negative symptoms, which helps you integrate into the community and ultimately achieve recovery.[25]

Important Points

- Family therapy improves your chances of staying in treatment, preventing relapse, and avoiding the need for hospitalization.
- Cognitive behavioral therapy helps you develop strategies to better cope with the symptoms your illness.

Conclusion

A major obstacle to recovery from schizophrenia is the underuse of effective psychological and behavioral approaches. We want to stress that integrating biological and psychological therapies to help you manage your symptoms is critical at all stages of this illness.[26] This chapter focuses on the psychological and behavioral approaches that demonstrate substantial benefit in both clinical studies and real-world settings. Just as with biological strategies, combining various psychological approaches can enhance your recovery.

5

Staying Well

People who have schizophrenia find it challenging to stay well—
to avoid experiencing a recurrence or worsening of their symptoms (referred to as a *relapse*). An essential part of preventing relapse is consistently taking antipsychotic medication, and one
of the biggest obstacles to staying well is the need to take medications daily. Although most people consider stopping their
medications at some point, doing so greatly increases the risk of
relapse and rehospitalization. Other keys to remaining well are
learning to manage stress; gaining insight into this condition,
which leads to self-acceptance; and coping with the stigma of
mental illness. This chapter explores these challenges as well as
strategies for managing them. As such, it is specifically addressed
to persons who have schizophrenia. As in the previous two chapters, however, family members and other loved ones will also
find useful information here (particularly the section "What Families Should Do").

Taking Medications

At least half of all people in the United States who are prescribed medications, regardless of their diagnosis, do not take them as prescribed. In schizophrenia, the most common reason for rehospitalization is stopping medications. Up to 50 percent of patients with schizophrenia relapse in the first year after remission (defined as having few or no symptoms), and more than 80 percent relapse by five years. People with schizophrenia who consistently take their medications, however, are less likely to need hospitalization.

Studies show that after multiple relapses, returning to the level of prior functioning, such as going to school or holding a job, becomes more difficult. Therefore, it is important to do everything possible to avoid relapse. Not taking medication as prescribed can range from missing a few *doses* of medication per week, to missing a few *days* of medication per week, to not taking medication at all. Relapses often happen when people who take their medication for several months start to feel better and begin to question the need to keep taking it. This lack of awareness or insight about their illness may be biological in origin, resulting from the brain changes associated with schizophrenia. You might say, "I feel fine, so why do I need the medication?" Ironically, it is not uncommon for people to forget that in most cases, they feel fine *because* of the medication. It is an important factor in helping them feel better and maintain wellness:

> Bob was 19 years old when he was first hospitalized for schizophrenia. He was convinced that his neighbors were working with the FBI to monitor him. According to him, this was part of a secret conspiracy to harm him in some way. He was hospitalized and started on antipsychotic medication, which helped him feel much better. Once again feeling comfortable in his neighborhood, he no longer believed that people were plotting against him. After about a year, he started to question whether he still needed

medication. He felt he was cured. He told his cousin, "There is nothing wrong with me."

Several weeks after Bob stopped his medication, his parents found him barricaded in the basement. Refusing to speak to them, he insisted on writing on a piece of paper: "I can't speak. They might hear me." Bob was subsequently hospitalized and restarted on his antipsychotic medication, with positive improvement in his condition.

Understanding the consequences of discontinuing medication, specifically the risk of having to return to the hospital, is helpful when you are tempted to stop taking yours. Not fully comprehending why you should continue taking your medication may not be the only reason you have for wanting to stop:

- *Denial.* You may wish you were not mentally ill, and the wish may be so strong that you decide you are not ill; hence there is no need to take medication.
- *Side effects from medication.* Akathisia (inner restlessness), akinesia (lack of spontaneous movement), sleepiness, and weight gain are particularly bothersome side effects of schizophrenia medications. For some people, additional medications are used to control the side effects of antipsychotics. Benztropine, for instance, is used to combat antipsychotic-induced EPS (*extrapyramidal side effects*, such as akathisia and akinesia). It is important to speak with your doctor about any side effects you are experiencing. A good approach is to bring a written list to the doctor's appointment detailing the suspected side effects, their frequency, and how long they have been troubling you.
- *Lack of trust in mental health care provider.* If you do not feel that your mental health care provider is listening to your concerns, then you might not take your medication. Cultural factors may also foster mistrust in the medical profession as a whole.

Research demonstrates that trust in the prescriber is key to ensuring that people take their medication. Trust is enhanced when the physician and patient work together as partners, rather than the doctor making decisions without any input from the patient. Whenever possible, you should share in decision making with your doctor. At appointments, you should feel free to express opinions about the medications so your doctor can integrate this information into the care plan.

Work with your doctor to find medications that minimize your side effects while maximally relieving your symptoms. A discussion with your doctor weighing the potential for benefits against the potential for side effects is a patient-centered approach that takes into account your individual values and beliefs.

- *Disorganized thinking* (forgetting or getting confused about medication). As discussed in chapter 1, disorganized thinking is common in schizophrenia and can hinder adherence to medication. You might completely forget the medication, or at the end of the day, you might not remember whether you took it, and because of this uncertainty, you could end up taking no medication that day. Your doctor should explain your medication to you during the office visit and provide written materials to help you understand how to take your medication and why it is being prescribed.

Making medication part of a daily routine, like brushing your teeth, can be helpful. It is important to take it at a convenient time each day (for instance, with breakfast or dinner). Studies show that the likelihood of a person taking his medication doubles with once-daily dosing compared with twice-daily dosing. Speak with your doctor about finding the simplest medication regimen, such as taking pills the fewest number of times per day, reducing the total number of medications, or switching to a once-daily medication. Pillboxes with separate compartments for different days and times of day can also be useful.

- *Hopelessness.* Schizophrenia is associated with depression, negativity, and loss of hope. If you see your situation as bleak, you may not feel like taking medication. Some individuals with schizophrenia believe that they will never get better or that "life is over" for them. This is not true. Although there is no cure, the illness can be successfully treated. To live the life that you want, you must fully engage in all aspects of treatment with your doctor and treatment team. The first step is to believe you can and will get better. A balanced life with meaningful relationships and stability is a realistic goal.

Probably the most common reason people with schizophrenia do not take their medications is the first reason we give above— the poor insight resulting from brain changes caused by their illness. They are not being stubborn and uncooperative, or lacking education about their condition. Rather, this lack of insight is the result of abnormal nerve functioning in the frontal lobes of the brain. This is the same area that may be responsible for hallucinations, delusions, and other symptoms of schizophrenia. Some experts believe that people with schizophrenia maintain a previous conception of themselves that reflects their higher functioning in the past (before they got sick), instead of how they are doing in the present.

Important Points
- There are many reasons people with schizophrenia might want to stop taking their medications.
- It is very important to speak with your doctor before stopping medication.

It can be useful to remember the benefits of taking medication. You should be encouraged to review these benefits with your mental health care provider or a family member. Making a list of pros and cons to medication can provide a balanced view. Finally, consider your medication in the context of your personal goals. In most cases, taking medication can help you reach your goals, whether this means living more independently, getting a job, maintaining a relationship, or going back to school.

Families can often tell when their loved ones have stopped taking their medications, because their symptoms get worse even though no stressful events or other triggers have occurred. In some instances, family members can count pills to document adherence. They can also play an important role in supporting a family member who needs to take medication, by providing words of encouragement and by personally observing the person take the medicine. Seeing a counselor or participating in a specialized support program can also be helpful.

The use of a once-monthly, long-acting injectable (LAI) medication may be preferable because it eliminates the need to remember to take a pill every day. In addition, an injection schedule provides more reliable information on what dosage of medication was received. Instead of having to remember to take a pill each day, you only have to remember to attend your appointment every month. Risk of rehospitalization may decrease with the use of LAI medications, which may also lead to better symptom control than pills. A recent formulation of LAI paliperidone only requires an injection every three months (four times a year).

For some people, additional support is required. Assertive community treatment (ACT) programs use case managers who visit patients in their homes to ensure adherence to doctors' appointments and medications. This was discussed in more detail in chapter 4.

Detecting the First Signs of Relapse

It is helpful to know the early signs that the illness is worsening. Although each person's experience is unique, some common early signs of relapse include:

- Insomnia or change in sleep patterns
- Problems with concentration
- Physical symptoms like headache, stomach pain, or increased heart rate
- Increased irritability and anger
- Feelings of fear or tension
- Decreased energy or fatigue
- Depressed mood

Once you know your personal relapse triggers, family members should be familiar with them as well, since your family may be the first to recognize the early signs of a relapse.

Preventing Relapse

Some people with schizophrenia feel better when they decide to ignore the voices they are hearing. Reminding yourself that the delusion is not true may also be helpful:

Jenny is 23 years old and has schizophrenia. Riding on the bus, she often thought that other people were talking about her. Once, two men in the seat behind her were laughing, and she was convinced that they were laughing at her. When this happened, Jenny stopped for a moment, closed her eyes, and remembered that this was just her "schizophrenia acting up." She reminded herself that her belief was not real, telling herself, "That is just my mind playing tricks on me. It isn't really happening."

Afterward, she felt calmer and was able to relax on the bus and think about other things. She labeled this her "self-talk" approach to "killing" the voices in her head.

The symptoms of schizophrenia may worsen when your mind is not occupied. Auditory hallucinations are loud and more distracting when you have nothing else to focus on. Delusional thinking, similarly, becomes more intense and distracting. Individuals with schizophrenia frequently state that when they are engaged in meaningful activities, their symptoms seem to fade into the background. Therefore, a key to staying well is to engage in activities *that are meaningful to you.* For some, this may be exercising, playing an instrument, or painting, while for others, it might be caring for a family member's children, cooking, or volunteering.

Martha is in her sixties and has schizophrenia. She used to spend all of her time sitting alone at home watching TV or just sitting on her bed. The voices in her head would get more distracting at these times. One day it got so bad that she decided she could not live like this anymore. She even contemplated suicide. When her sister invited her to join her weekly bridge group, Martha hesitated at first. With some encouragement, she decided to give it a try. Soon, she began to look forward to the weekly get-together. Her mood brightened because she had something meaningful to look forward to every week. The voices did not seem to bother her much when she focused on her bridge group.

Pursuing interests improves self-esteem, promotes self-reliance, and allows your mind to focus on things other than hallucinations or paranoid ideas. Being engaged in outside activities also lifts the mood and prevents depression and loneliness, both of which interfere with taking antipsychotic medications.

Joining a self-help group can also be beneficial. Schizophrenia is a very lonely illness, and knowing that you are not alone in your struggles can be reassuring. The National Alliance on Mental Illness (NAMI) provides resources, including support groups. Schizophrenics Anonymous and Psychosis Free are national groups focused on providing education and support for people who have schizophrenia.

Maintaining a healthy lifestyle can also help you stay well. Getting enough sleep (eight hours per night) and eating a balanced diet are important. It's best to avoid large amounts of fast food, fried food, and junk food like chips, candy, and cookies. The focus should be on eating lean meats like chicken and turkey; fish; fruits and vegetables; whole grains like granola and whole wheat bread; and beans. Regular exercise is also advised. Go walking every day, join a gym, swim, or do yoga. All are beneficial for both mind and body.

Substance abuse is a common cause of relapse. Many abused drugs affect the parts of the brain that are disrupted by schizophrenia and, as a result, can cause symptoms that resemble this disorder. Marijuana may seem to have a calming effect, but in most people, it actually worsens paranoia. Cocaine can cause hallucinations that resemble schizophrenia. Use of these and other drugs frequently cause relapse. If you are using these drugs, you should work with your doctor to obtain appropriate specialized treatment. Untreated depression or anxiety may also interfere with adherence and lead to relapse.

Managing Stress

Stress is a frequent trigger for relapse. Major life occurrences, such as the death of a loved one, moving, or getting a divorce are stressful for nearly everyone. Chronic, persistent stressors might include living in an unsafe neighborhood, not having enough money to pay rent, or repeated arguments with friends or loved ones. Managing stress, therefore, is essential to staying well.

The first step is identifying the people, places, or situations that you find stressful. For some, this might be having to spend time with a large number of people, such as at a family reunion. In this case, you might decide to spend smaller amounts of time with family members, with planned moments away from the group to avoid feeling overwhelmed. Situations with a lot of stimuli, such as being around many people talking at the same time, may feel confusing and elicit paranoia or other psychotic symptoms. Schizophrenia involves problems with information processing, so high-stimulation situations may "overload" you. When you know that a demanding time is coming, think ahead and make a plan so that you can get everything done in an adequate amount of time. Eating a balanced diet and exercising also help to maintain regular sleep patterns, which can decrease auditory hallucinations and help with managing stress.

Having a regular routine and schedule is useful for many people with schizophrenia. A daily routine provides structure and a sense of regularity that reduces unpredictability and surprises. This will allow you to anticipate stresses and potentially destabilizing events. Situations that are unexpected are often the most difficult to tolerate.

Insight: Accepting Your Illness

Persons newly diagnosed with diabetes may tell their doctor, "I do not have diabetes. You are wrong. I don't think it is true." This happens despite lab work and blood sugar values that clearly indicate diabetes. The desire to not have the illness is so strong that they deny reality. The same can be true of schizophrenia.

Accepting the illness is the first step to mastering it. We want to be defined by our accomplishments, not our diagnosis. Once you accept treatment, then the symptoms can be appropriately addressed so that they recede into the background, and you can go on living your life. This will enable you to be in control rather than the illness. Controlling the symptoms prevents you from being defined by the illness, so you can live life as you want and be someone who just happens to have schizophrenia.

What Families Should Do

How best to respond to an individual who lacks insight has been an intense area of research. It can be frustrating trying to work with someone who is not accepting help. Being supportive works better than lecturing people about their illness. Acceptance of a diagnosis such as schizophrenia can be a long process, and each person does it at her own speed. Above all, family members should listen to their loved one. Try not to argue with the person; just respect her point of view. Focus on trying to understand without necessarily agreeing or disagreeing. Convey comprehension of her experience and all the reasons she has for not taking her medications. Look for points where you and your relative see things the same way.

Melvin, 31 years old, has been hospitalized eleven times since age 19 for auditory hallucinations telling him to take an overdose of his pills. He is convinced that the FBI is monitoring him. Since the FBI is doing this and not him, he does not understand why he has to take medication. His sister, Glenda, insists that he see a doctor every month, but Melvin refuses, telling her, "I am fine. Leave me alone." He did not view himself as ill. His point of view was different from hers. Glenda felt she had to pester Melvin to take medication for his schizophrenia. She would confront her brother about it, but that only seemed to drive him away.

This went on for a year, and Melvin was hospitalized again twice in that time. After realizing that nagging and fighting did not work, Glenda changed her approach. She no longer brought up his illness and stopped using the term "schizophrenia," because Melvin did not think that he was sick. Instead she just listened to him nonjudgmentally, which was very hard at first. In an effort to understand him better, she tried to put herself in his place: "So Melvin, it sounds like you feel you are okay now and that you don't need medications." Though this was hard for her to say, Melvin started to engage with her in a more positive way. He described how the medications made him feel "slowed down" and that he felt everyone was "pushing pills" on him even though, he said, "I'm not crazy." Instead of challenging him, Glenda simply tried to understand her brother.

Glenda's initial focus was on her brother being "ill" and having a condition that needed medication. After changing her approach, she asked Melvin what he wanted for his life. He revealed that he wanted to attend a nearby community college, just as Glenda had done years ago. In fact, Melvin had enrolled in this school several times in the past but had dropped out each time when he got too paranoid. Glenda and her brother discussed this pattern. Melvin was able to see that he usually had to drop out of school after he stopped his medication. From that time on, the focus for Glenda and Melvin changed to how the medications helped Melvin reach a goal (staying in school). No longer was the focus on being ill, "being schizophrenic," or what others felt was best for him. After a few years, Melvin was able to get his associate degree in criminal justice at a local community college.

This common-sense approach has been summarized by the acronym LEAP: listen, empathize, agree, and partner (see the reference by Xavier Amador at the end of this chapter). Family members should *listen* nonjudgmentally and try to understand the feelings (*empathize*) of their relative without arguing or judging. *Agree* refers to finding points that everyone can agree on. Glenda did not agree that Melvin did not need medication or that he was not sick. But the two did agree that medications helped him stay in school. From that point on, they worked as *partners* in his treatment rather than as adversaries.

Stigma

Stigma refers to a negative attitude or belief about a particular group, in this case, people with schizophrenia. This frequently stems from negative stereotypes in movies and on television. People with schizophrenia are portrayed as dangerous and scary and therefore to be feared or avoided. Stigma is a frequent obstacle to taking medication. Because of fear of stigma, friends or family members may tell you not to take psychiatric medications.

> Susan has had schizophrenia for the last three years. When her brother told her, "You shouldn't take those medications; only crazy people take medications," Susan stopped taking them. Weeks later, she was taken to the local emergency room by police officers who found her wandering the streets, mumbling to herself. She was subsequently hospitalized and restarted on her medications.

Family members need to acknowledge and address their own negative stereotypes about schizophrenia. They may incorrectly advise you to just "be strong" or "pray and it will go away." While positive thinking and religious faith may help in recovery, on their own they are not an adequate treatment for schizophrenia. Self-stigma refers to when people with schizophrenia, like you, stop their medications because of their own internal shame and fears of being viewed as "weak," "defective," or "a basket case." You are not weak or defective, but you do have a medical condition that requires treatment with medication.

For family members and friends, stigma toward people with schizophrenia can be overcome by becoming educated about the condition. Reading this book is a good start. Learning about how the disorder can be treated demystifies it and reduces the negative associations with having schizophrenia. Talking to mental health professionals or attending a peer support group is also useful. Hearing the stories of other people with schizophrenia who have achieved their goals (for example, going to school or raising children) may help you see your loved one's true potential and diminish stigmatizing feelings. Help him see that he is a worthwhile person. This creates a sense of hope for the future. Knowing that a family member believes in him helps develop self-esteem and confidence to work toward future goals.

Important Points

- Not taking antipsychotic medication as prescribed is the most common reason for relapse and rehospitalization.
- There are numerous reasons for discontinuing medication, including a feeling of hopelessness, lack of trust in providers, and disorganized thinking. Lack of disease insight because of the brain illness of schizophrenia is the most common cause.
- The LEAP method is a useful approach to poor insight: Listen to your loved one. Empathize with her, find areas to Agree on, and Partner on connecting her life goals to taking medication.
- Other approaches to staying well include maintaining a healthy lifestyle, managing stress, and overcoming stigma.

RESOURCES

Amador, X. *I Am Not Sick, I Don't Need Help*. New York: Vida Press, 2012. Helpful guide for family members working with a relative who is refusing treatment.

National Alliance on Mental Illness (NAMI). www.nami.org. NAMI's "In Our Own Voice" video challenges stereotypes about mental illness. This site also provides information about local peer-to-peer support groups that help adults with mental illness better understand their condition.

Schizophrenia and Related Disorders Alliance of America (SARDAA). www.sardaa.org. Schizophrenics Anonymous, a self-help organization, can be reached through SARDAA. The website offers information and stories about people who are recovering from schizophrenia.

Treatment Advocacy Center. www.treatmentadvocacycenter.org. This website focuses on eliminating barriers to mental health treatment, including related legal issues.

6

Schizophrenia and the Family

Family members play an essential role in improving the lives of people with schizophrenia. They are a valuable source of emotional support and practical help. Understandably, being a family member of someone who has schizophrenia often brings significant challenges. Communication within the family may be difficult, and relationships may change or suffer for everyone in the family. This chapter specifically addresses family members and explores the range of emotions that people experience when their loved one has schizophrenia. We also discuss coping methods and practical strategies for parents, siblings, and children of people who have schizophrenia.

Expanding Role for Family Members

Through the 1960s, many people with schizophrenia remained hospitalized for years in large government-supported psychiatric institutions. In that era of long-term hospitalizations, families played a relatively small role in the patient's daily life. Later in the twentieth century, however, individuals with schizophrenia moved out into the community, as antipsychotic medications were developed, and the trend toward releasing people with schizophrenia from hospitals gained momentum. In this new era, family members became more engaged in their loved one's life, playing an active role in that person's day-to-day care. Unfortunately, the U.S. health care system does not always provide adequate support for family members who take on these expanded responsibilities.

As a family member, you may take on multiple roles to help the person with schizophrenia—including case manager, cook, maid, accountant, nurse, and counselor—all at the same time. These roles are generally time consuming, and they affect family members in a variety of ways:

- *Loss of personal time.* Your days may be monopolized by the ill person, so you no longer have time for your normal daily activities.
- *Fewer social relationships.* You may have less time and energy to devote to maintaining friendships.
- *Poorer health status.* Your own health needs may be neglected as you devote increasing amounts of time to playing other roles.
- *Loss of income.* You may be forced to quit a job or reduce your hours at work so that you can care for the ill person.

As we discuss later in this chapter, family care providers must always take care of themselves and make sure their own needs are met; otherwise, they will not likely be able to help the person with schizophrenia for the long term. Getting additional support for the person who has schizophrenia and getting education, training, and counseling for themselves will make a world of difference for everyone.

Communication

Many families ask, *"How should I behave toward someone who has schizophrenia?"* Happily, the answer is straightforward: treat the person with kindness and respect—exactly how you would want to be treated. In most cases, the person wants to be treated like everyone else.

Another common question is, *"What's the best way to talk to a person who has schizophrenia?"* It's best to communicate with the person in brief, clear statements. There are no specific topics to avoid. Schizophrenia affects a person's ability to process a large amount of stimuli—or information—at one time. People who have schizophrenia can easily become overwhelmed in large gatherings or other settings where many sounds and images are coming at them all at once.

People with schizophrenia may also be impaired in their ability to process information in seemingly simple conversations. It may take time for your loved one to comprehend the information, so you may need to be patient, and you may need to repeat. It's best to pose one question at a time and repeat or rephrase the question if you sense that repetition might be helpful.

"What should I do when my family member exhibits delusional thinking?" You may be inclined to argue, or to point out how his thinking is incorrect. This is usually not a useful approach. When the person who has schizophrenia insists that the delusion is accurate, he may even ask you to confirm that you agree with him. In this case, it may be best to acknowledge how the person feels while stating that you do not see it the same way that he does:

Barbara was seeing snakes coming up from the sidewalk. She told her brother, Bob, that the snakes were being sent up from the devil to "make my life hell." She insisted this was happening. Bob would point at the sidewalk and say, "You see, there are no snakes there." Bob's statements irritated Barbara and made her focus more on the snakes. Finally, Bob realized that arguing with her was not getting anywhere. Instead he told her, "I know you believe there are snakes coming from the sidewalk, but let's just see if we can keep walking."

While Bob did not reinforce that her delusion was true, he was still able to validate Barbara's experience. Avoid responding to delusional thoughts with sarcastic or supposedly "humorous" responses (such as saying, in a sarcastic tone, "Oh yes, Barbara, there are huge snakes coming up from the sidewalk, *for sure!*"); such responses tend to confuse the individual and may reinforce the delusion.

Schizophrenia can make the back and forth exchange of conversation very difficult. Many families are concerned about what they should do if the person with schizophrenia appears aloof and uninterested in discussions. First, you should not take this behavior personally, because it is most often due, at least in part, to the nature of the illness. Second, if your family member appears withdrawn and isolates herself from others, it may be better to leave her be. She is likely to be listening to the conversations taking place around her even when she is not able to participate. Many people who have schizophrenia find it hard to express their feelings to others. Limiting the size of social gatherings can be helpful. Third, keep in mind that the person may feel better spending time alone, and that withdrawing from situations may be a way of coping with overstimulating experiences. If the withdrawal becomes severe or persistent, it may signal an impending worsening of the illness. In this case, family members should be supportive and guide the person into mental health treatment.

It is well known that individuals with schizophrenia are particularly sensitive to environmental stress. Situational frustration may lead to communication patterns within families that are intense and counterproductive. Such an unfavorable family environment is referred to as *expressed emotion,* or EE. Emotional overinvolvement, hostility, and critical comments directed toward the ill person are characteristics of EE. Research has shown that EE in family interactions increases the chances of relapse in patients with schizophrenia. The following sections explain how to minimize these adverse types of interactions.

Feelings of Family Members

Most people who have schizophrenia rely on their family members for a great deal of help. In addition to emotional support, a lot of practical support is given, such as cooking, cleaning, managing finances, and organizing doctors' appointments. Much of this help is given every day. Few people who are providing this level of support can avoid feeling that their usual lives and routines are being encroached on by having to care for the ill person. The behavior of the person with schizophrenia may be unpredictable and hard to manage, frequently straining relationships. Bizarre behavior may be bewildering and even frightening to family members: putting glue in one's hair, walking outside in the middle of the night, or hiding in the basement because of a conviction that the government is monitoring every move. Negative symptoms, such as sitting in front of a blank TV screen for hours or not bathing, can be equally frustrating.

A range of feelings are experienced by people whose loved one has schizophrenia:

- *Despair and sadness.* Having these feelings for the affected relative is not uncommon. Along with these feelings come general worry and distress, hopelessness, and negative feelings about the future.
- *Frustration.* Family members caring for an ill loved one often feel undervalued. You may feel unrecognized and unappreciated by the medical system and not adequately

involved in medical decision making. Frustration may also stem from feeling that you and your loved one are not able to access all the mental health services that he needs.

- *Guilt.* Parents of an person with schizophrenia may feel guilt for neglecting other children. You may find yourself spending an inordinate amount of time focusing on the care of your affected child. Meanwhile, your other children receive less attention. Most people also feel torn by other responsibilities, such as a full-time job or caring for elderly parents, who also demand and need time and attention. As a parent, you may blame yourself for your child's schizophrenia. Some parents feel they could have prevented the disease if they had somehow treated their child differently, *but this is rarely the case.* Finally, you may feel guilt over not recognizing the symptoms sooner. John remembers how he first felt when his daughter Lisa was diagnosed: "I thought that there must have been something that my wife and I did wrong. How could this disease have just happened? Maybe I was too strict with her. There is some mental illness that runs in my family, so I am probably to blame in the end."

- *Feelings of loss.* Many people feel they have "lost" their loved one to the disease of schizophrenia, because that person no longer seems to be who he once was. Maria recounts how her son, Luis, changed after becoming ill: "Luis was popular in high school. He excelled at sports and was captain of the football team. He had plans to go to college. Now that he has schizophrenia, he just sits around the house all day. He rarely says anything, though sometimes he will mumble out loud when no one is there. He doesn't play football or talk to any of his friends. I feel like I lost the son I once had. I don't know this person."

- *Shame and embarrassment.* Family members may feel the stigma of mental illness leading to shame. You may feel shunned by friends and neighbors, and you may feel socially isolated and sad.

- *Fear of developing schizophrenia.* The children of someone who has schizophrenia may worry that they will develop schizophrenia themselves. Siblings of the person with schizophrenia may have the same worry.
- *Fatigue and anger.* The demands of everyday caregiving can cause anger and resentment. You may ask yourself, *"Why did this have to happen to her? Why did this happen to my family?"* You may have to make sacrifices in your career when you are forced to work reduced hours or to retire early to care for your loved one. These sacrifices may in turn lead to financial difficulties for the household. It's not unusual to feel angry over the disruption in normal family and social life that happens because the family has to care for the ill individual.

Strategies for Families

You are a highly valuable source of practical and emotional support for your loved one who has schizophrenia. It is often a family member who is the first to get the person into treatment. When families are involved in seeking help, the individual spends less time untreated.

Recognizing your own value is important, but that recognition may not provide much help in dealing with the unexpected frustrations and challenges of living with a person who has schizophrenia. In the following sections, we discuss some strategies for coping and for helping your loved one, yourself, and the rest of your family.

Education

Learning about schizophrenia is essential to managing it. Reading a book like this one and other books and articles can provide a framework for understanding the illness. In-person professional psychoeducation, which is focused on teaching patients and families about the illness, can be very helpful. Psychoeducation services are provided by mental health organizations across the country, such as National Alliance on Mental Illness (NAMI), and are led by professionals or trained relatives of people who have mental illness. Programs such as NAMI's "Family to Family" have increased understanding about mental illness, improved families' ability to solve problems, reduced stress, and improved acceptance of the family member's illness.

Support Adherence to Treatment

Many people who have schizophrenia have a poor understanding or awareness of their illness. They may seem unbothered by having no friends or job. People who have poor self-insight are harder to help because, for example, they may not accept the need to take prescribed medications. Individuals who do not take prescribed antipsychotics and other medications may have more symptom episodes, emergency room visits, and hospitalizations. Guidance provided by a family member can often make the difference in people getting the treatment they need and taking the medications that help them, which in turn helps the family avoid crises and time spent in the ER.

Research shows that having an available and supportive family helps people with schizophrenia adhere to treatment. Individuals may be symptomatic (experiencing hallucinations, feeling paranoid, and so on) but not think they need to take any medication for their schizophrenia. This can be extremely frustrating for the family member who is trying to help. Your loved one may become argumentative if you or other family members push medications too hard. It is best to state clearly why you think medications make a difference (for example, "You seem so much happier and more relaxed when you're taking your medication"), rather than to constantly nag the person about it. In many cases, it is helpful for the family member to "be in charge" of giving the medication to the person each day. Not only does this help remind her to take the medication, but it can also *confirm* that the medication is actually being taken. People with schizophrenia who do not have a supportive and present family are more likely to disengage with treatment and stop taking their medications. The American Psychiatric Association treatment guidelines for schizophrenia endorse the role of family to improve outcomes in schizophrenia. As noted above, the family's involvement often increases when psychosis is worsening and the person is in need of higher levels of support.

Families of mentally ill persons have expressed frustration with their ability to access the mental health system. Many family members wish for increased involvement and contact with their loved one's psychiatrist. Such involvement helps reduce stress within the family unit and can provide reassurance to the family. Developing trust in the mental health professional to establish a good relationship should be a priority for most families. Ideally, the family works in collaboration with the treatment team to maximize recovery. You will find support by maintaining regular contact with the psychiatrist. Ask for regular updates and the next steps in treatment. You, in turn, can also provide valuable insight to the psychiatrist regarding how your loved one is doing. In most states, however, the ill person must sign a release of information to allow family members to speak to their physician. The patient's physician may be willing to help you talk with your loved one about the need for him to sign the release and about how helpful communication among the patient, the physician, and the family can be.

Recognize the First Signs of Relapse

Do you know how to recognize the first signs of impending decline in your loved one's health? As we discuss in chapter 5, potential signs of relapse include disrupted sleep, change in mood, increased social isolation, and decreased ability to handle stress.

Encourage Independence

It may be best to allow the ill person to have a room of her own in the home. This allows her to have a quiet place to be alone. You may also have to decide the degree of independence allowed to your loved one. A good approach is to allow her to be as independent as possible while maintaining personal safety. For instance, the person is permitted more independence (such as driving to the store alone) once certain other safeguards are in place (such as demonstrating that she knows the route to the store by heart, remembers to lock the car doors, remembers to wear a seatbelt, and so on). The ability to manage money varies among individuals; some people with schizophrenia need a family member to handle finances. Allowing the person to handle some money, such as a weekly allowance, may help her feel more independent and develop better money-handling skills. Having the expectation that she will perform regular household chores also encourages independence and raises self-esteem.

Identify Strengths

Try to point out to the person with schizophrenia the things he is doing well. Commend him for keeping his doctors' appointments or taking his medication. Remarking on how nicely he is dressed or how clean he smells can encourage better hygiene. Sharon, who has schizophrenia, describes how such an interaction with her husband encouraged her:

> I have always loved to cook. Even before I became ill, people always told me how much they loved my lasagna. After I became ill, it was hard for me to concentrate on cooking; the recipes seemed too complicated. When my husband reminded me how

much he loved my cooking, it gave me the courage to try it again. It was hard at first to follow some of the recipes, but I am now able to cook many of the dishes that I made in the past. I feel good when my family tells me that they like what I made for dinner.

Reduce Stress and Overstimulation in the Home Environment

Family interventions focused on reducing expressed emotion (EE, that hostile environment discussed earlier in the chapter) are beneficial. Learning to communicate without hostility or criticism is key.

Maintain Routines and Consistency

Maintaining structure within the household is important, because a predictable schedule is reassuring to the person with schizophrenia. "House rules" help to define which behaviors are unacceptable. Examples of disallowed behaviors may include verbal threats and physical violence. Regular bathing may be a requirement in some households, while other families may focus more on household chores being regularly completed.

Make Sure Your Own Needs Are Met

It may be tempting at times to completely take over the life of the person with mental illness. Not only is this impossible, it is not a good long-term approach for the person as she works to become more independent, or for you, because you will feel increasingly overburdened.

Get Support When Needed

It is okay to ask for help. In addition to seeking support from the ill person's psychiatrist, you may find it beneficial to obtain individual counseling for yourself. This is an excellent way to process the feelings of your own experience separate from your affected family member.

Support Long-Term Recovery

Family therapy can help reduce relapse rates. Talk to your loved one's psychiatrist to learn more about family-focused approaches that can help reduce the burden on caregivers like you and improve overall family functioning. These approaches focus on minimizing disruption to the family unit and resolving feelings of grief, stress, and resentment.

Intensive skills training may also be available for relatives. These programs last up to nine months and employ cognitive behavioral techniques focused on coaching, prompting, modeling, and problem-solving skills. Unfortunately, these programs are not widely available in all parts of the country.

Violence

Although anger is fairly common in people with schizophrenia, most people with this disorder are not physically violent. Most of the small number of individuals who become violent are abusing drugs or are not taking their antipsychotic medications. This is another reason that taking medications, on schedule, is so important. As with anger or other strong emotions, the urge to become violent may be rooted in psychotic symptoms the person is experiencing, such as paranoia, delusions of being controlled, or delusions of reference (the belief discussed in chapter 1 that outside objects have a special meaning to the person). There may also be command hallucinations: for instance, a voice may be telling the person with schizophrenia to hurt a specific person in order to save the world. Violence may also result from anger that is rooted in feelings of sadness, stress, and frustration.

It is important to identify and acknowledge the person's under-lying feelings. Sit down with your family member to talk about what is making him angry, and try to work out together the rea-sons behind his anger. The long list of potential issues that might be bothering someone with schizophrenia include:

- Misunderstanding another person's emotions or motives
- Discomfort or fear about a social situation
- Feeling criticized or made fun of by others
- Anger related to physical pain or poor physical health
- Disappointment about being unable to meet expectations

Once your loved one can say out loud what is bothering him, the situation may be diffused, and physical violence may be avoided. By talking with the person, you may identify a misunderstanding that is causing him to feel this way.

The three most common risk factors for violent behavior are al-cohol and drug abuse, not taking medication, and having been vi-olent in the past. The best approach for families is to be aware of warning signs of impending violent activity and to take steps to prevent it. For instance, it may be best to keep guns or other weap-ons and sharp knives locked up when there is a history of violent behavior. It may be necessary to convey clear consequences for al-cohol or drug abuse as way to deter the person from this behavior. If there is an immediate threat of violence, it is important to remain calm and allow the person lots of space (remain physically distant from him). Do not hesitate to call the police if you feel you or your loved ones are in danger.

When Your Loved One Is Thinking about Suicide

People who have schizophrenia have a higher risk of committing suicide than people in the general population. If you are a family member of someone who talks about committing suicide or who makes a suicide attempt, you understandably find it very disturbing to know that your loved one wants to end her life.

The factors that are associated with a higher risk of suicide include a history of previous suicide attempts, being socially isolated, feeling sad or hopeless, experiencing an increase in auditory hallucinations or delusions, and using drugs or alcohol. People who have schizophrenia may also commit suicide as a reaction to realizing how severe their illness is. This is particularly true for individuals who were previously high achieving and then lost their ability to function at a high level after becoming ill.

Family members need to know the signs that the person may be suicidal, which are:

- Feeling down or blue
- Being preoccupied with death or dying
- Making statements like "I might as well die" or "There's no point in living." It is particularly concerning if the person has a specific plan for how she would commit suicide.
- Expressing inconsolable guilt
- Making a will, giving away valued possessions, or similar acts
- Hearing voices that are harsh or critical
- Hearing voices telling her to hurt herself

Always encourage the person to open up about *any* feelings she has, including suicidal thoughts. Asking someone if she is having thoughts of harming herself will not "give" her the idea. Rather, it will make it acceptable for her to talk about it. If a person can learn to share her feelings early on with a loved one, then in many instances, the urges can be addressed before they become overwhelming. If your family member does become suicidal, however, remember these basic principles:

1. Be supportive. Try to respond openly to your loved one's concerns, and express support. Do not ignore what she is

saying or be judgmental. Point out the reasons that she should not take her own life.
2. Explore with the person how she is feeling, what she is thinking about, and whether she has made a specific plan to commit suicide.
3. Whenever possible, remove any potential weapons or sharp objects from the home. Do not let the person out of your sight.
4. Maintain open communication, as it may be comforting for the person to freely express herself.
5. If the individual has attempted suicide in the past or is expressing a plan to hurt herself, then she should be immediately evaluated by a medical professional. Either take the person to the nearest emergency room (ER) or call 911.
6. If you are uncertain what to do, then it is always a safe choice to get your loved one to an ER for an evaluation. Contacting a suicide hotline can provide additional help. See the resources at the end of this chapter.

Important Points

- Family members play an essential role in the lives of individuals with schizophrenia.
- Feelings of anger, frustration, sadness, fatigue, and shame are common and expected among people who are dealing with a relative who has schizophrenia.
- Support your loved one in any way possible but be aware of the limits of your ability to help. Stay alert for the signs indicating that your relative is getting sicker, and help him get the needed care; encourage the person to take his medication regularly; highlight his strengths whenever possible and help him stay on track toward his goals.

Conclusion

Families play an important caregiving role for persons with schizophrenia. This role may affect many areas of the family members' lives. It is common for family members to have strong emotions, some of which are negative, as a result of having responsibilities for someone with schizophrenia. Strategies for supporting family members cope with this situation on a daily basis can be helpful to the entire family, including the person who has schizophrenia.

RESOURCES

National Alliance on Mental Illness (NAMI). www.nami.org.
National Institute of Mental Health (NIMH). www.nimh.nih.gov.
National Institute of Mental Health. "Schizophrenia." Last revised May 2020. www.nimh.nih.gov/health/topics/schizophrenia/index.shtml.
Schizophrenia.com. www.schizophrenia.com.

7

Medical Conditions and Schizophrenia

You may be concerned about your loved one's physical health. Your sister or brother, parent or child, may be overweight, out of shape, or not take good care of himself or herself. People with schizophrenia are more likely than other people to suffer from a number of medical conditions, including heart disease, obesity, and diabetes. There are several explanations for this. One is that some people who have schizophrenia tend to eat a lot of junk food and do not get enough exercise, both of which contribute to the development of disease. Lack of access to medical treatment, or inadequate treatment of common medical conditions, can also be factors. In addition, the side effects of certain medications may contribute to the development of these conditions.

This chapter focuses on what you as a family member can do to help your loved one to stay healthy. As such, much of the information will also be directly useful to the person with schizophrenia. We review the medical conditions that people with schizophrenia may have and explain how better screening, prevention, and treatment of these conditions can lead to better health.

Medical Problems that Are More Common in People Who Have Schizophrenia

Studies show that people with schizophrenia are more likely to develop asthma, chronic obstructive pulmonary disease (COPD, or emphysema), diabetes mellitus, hepatitis C, coronary artery disease, and congestive heart failure. Your relative might complain of feeling short of breath or having chest pain, both of which are common complaints among those with schizophrenia. These findings are true in the United States and in the countries of Europe and Asia.

Even more concerning is that people with schizophrenia die younger than the average person in the United States. Several studies report death rates that are four to eight times higher than people of the same age who do not have schizophrenia. Studies show that men with schizophrenia die sooner than women with the disorder. In most cases, the primary reason for dying earlier is heart disease, though cancer has also been identified as a significant cause of death. Schizophrenia is associated with a lifespan that is 20 percent, or about one-fifth, shorter than the average lifespan. To put it another way, if the average person dies at age 76, then the average person with schizophrenia dies at 61. Most of these lost years of life are taken by heart disease. Suicide accounts for a smaller but still important number of deaths—about 10 to 15 percent of people with schizophrenia take their own lives.

Why does heart disease have such a significant negative effect on the lives of people with schizophrenia? One reason is that individuals with schizophrenia suffer from an unusually high number of risk factors for heart disease. For instance, your loved one may have gained a lot of weight and may now be obese; he may sit on the couch all day and not move around much, or he may smoke and have high cholesterol or diabetes. Compounding the problem is that these heart disease risk factors are frequently not detected or treated.

Medical Care of People Who Have Schizophrenia

Do you know the last time your loved one went to see her primary care doctor? There is a good chance that she has not seen a doctor for general medical care in a very long time, if ever. Poor quality health care and lack of access to health care are common, challenging, and significant problems for persons who have schizophrenia. Studies have shown that poor health care contributes to higher death rates in people with the disorder. For instance, studies in Ireland and Finland found that in both countries, an increased likelihood of dying was linked to poor medical care and disconnection from the health services that would have adequately addressed their medical conditions.

People with schizophrenia often have a difficult time accessing health care. Compared with those who have other mental illnesses, people with schizophrenia are less likely to have a primary care physician and more likely to have trouble seeing a doctor. Those with diabetes or hypertension in addition to schizophrenia have significantly fewer medical visits than those who have diabetes or hypertension but do not have schizophrenia. When individuals with schizophrenia and either diabetes or hypertension were questioned about their health care, they identified the following barriers to care:

- Providers did not take their health complaints seriously.
- Nonpsychiatrists were reluctant to provide them with comprehensive care.
- The patients were not offered screening procedures.

If your relative does not regularly see a doctor, he may have a medical condition that he does not know about. Underdiagnosis of everyday medical conditions is a common problem. Elevated rates of undiagnosed (and therefore untreated) high blood pressure, elevated cholesterol, and high blood sugar have been reported even in hospitalized patients with schizophrenia (that is, people who were clearly receiving medical care and being seen by medical professionals). Even when people with schizophrenia are in regular contact with doctors or other health care professionals, they are less likely to have their cancer or heart disease diagnosed.

When a medical diagnosis is made, does your loved one receive the appropriate treatment for his medical condition? The Clinical Antipsychotic Trials of Intervention Effectiveness (CATIE) Study compared various antipsychotic medications in a group of more than 1,400 patients with schizophrenia. Rates of diabetes, hypertension, and hyperlipidemia (elevated cholesterol) were higher in people with schizophrenia than in those without psychiatric illness. A study of individuals with schizophrenia found that up to 30 percent of those with diabetes were not receiving treatment, while nearly 90 percent with hypertension were not receiving treatment. These are surprisingly high rates, particularly given that all the patients were receiving regular psychiatric care. Some studies, though not all, show that heart disease in particular is managed differently in these patients. For instance, adults with schizophrenia hospitalized for a heart attack are less likely to receive cardiac catheterization (a procedure to evaluate blood flow to the heart), percutaneous transluminal angioplasty (a procedure to open up blocked arteries), or life-saving coronary artery bypass graft (CABG) surgery.

Screening

Screening for common medical conditions also occurs at lower rates in people with schizophrenia. Compared with people who do not have schizophrenia of the same age and gender, those who have the disorder have fewer medical visits and are less likely to receive a detailed physical exam, lipid screening, or colon cancer screening. Women with schizophrenia are less likely to receive a Papanicolaou (Pap) smear, a standard screening procedure for early detection of cervical cancer.

Specific Medical Conditions

Hypertension

Hypertension, a condition of elevated blood pressure, poses a significant risk for heart disease. Among people with hypertension, those who also have schizophrenia are 40 percent more likely to die. In the large CATIE trial, one-third of patients were found to have high blood pressure; and other large studies have found similarly elevated rates. In addition, treatment with a second-generation antipsychotic (such as olanzapine, risperidone, or quetiapine) is associated with elevated blood pressure. (The side effects of antipsychotics related to weight gain are described later in this chapter.) It is important to note, however, that not all studies have found increased rates of hypertension in people who have schizophrenia.

The ideal blood pressure is lower than 120/80 mm Hg for persons of all ages. Appropriate medications for treatment of hypertension include thiazide-type diuretics (a type of water pill), such as hydrochlorothiazide or chlorthalidone; angiotensin-converting enzyme (ACE) inhibitors, such as lisinopril or enalapril; angiotensin receptor blockers, such as losartan or valsartan; or calcium channel blockers, such as amlodipine. A low salt diet and exercise are recommended for everyone with elevated blood pressure.

Elevated Cholesterol

Has your family member or friend with schizophrenia had her cholesterol checked? Individuals with schizophrenia are more likely to have elevated cholesterol (hyperlipidemia), another important risk factor for heart disease. Studies show an increased risk of heart disease from hyperlipidemia. Like elevated blood pressure, elevated cholesterol has been associated with the use of second-generation antipsychotics. Everyone with elevated cholesterol should eat a low-fat diet, avoiding deep-fried foods and red meat, and eating more vegetables and high-fiber foods). Many people with high cholesterol require treatment with statin medications, such as atorvastatin or rosuvastatin to lower cholesterol levels in the blood.

Obesity, Metabolic Syndrome, and Diabetes Mellitus

Your loved one has likely gained some weight since becoming ill or starting medications. For many reasons, individuals with schizophrenia are more likely to be obese. Eating a healthy diet and exercising regularly may prevent or reverse obesity. Negative symptoms and cognitive impairment in schizophrenia (as discussed in chapter 1) result in decreased motivation to eat well and exercise. As a consequence, people with schizophrenia are more likely to follow an unhealthy diet (for example, eating too much fast food and soft drinks while not eating enough fruits and vegetables) and less likely to exercise. These lifestyle habits increase their risk of developing obesity and elevated blood sugar. Further, their psychiatric medications may make them tired or sleepy, which interferes with leading an active lifestyle.

Metabolic syndrome refers to a group of risk factors that, when occurring together, greatly increase the risk for diabetes and heart disease. This syndrome is more common in people with schizophrenia. The diagnosis of metabolic syndrome requires three of five criteria:

1. Waist circumference ≥ 40 inches (men) or ≥ 35 inches (women)
2. Fasting triglycerides ≥ 150 mg/dl

3. High density lipoprotein (HDL) ≤ 40 mg/dl (men) or ≤ 50 mg/dl (women)
4. Blood pressure ≥ 135/85 mm Hg
5. Fasting blood glucose ≥ 110 mg/dl

Diabetes is a disorder of the hormone insulin that leads to elevated blood sugar. A person who has diabetes is more likely to develop heart disease. Schizophrenia is associated with increased rates of elevated blood sugar and diabetes. Some research shows this association even in people with schizophrenia who are not taking an antipsychotic medication, but antipsychotics are known to increase the risk of elevated blood sugar and diabetes. Diabetes may lead to several life-threatening complications, including kidney failure (often requiring hemodialysis), foot amputation, stroke, and blindness. All of these are preventable if diabetes is diagnosed and treated early in its course. Elevated blood sugar levels confirm the diagnosis. Initial treatment includes lifestyle changes (exercise and dietary changes) and a medication called metformin. Some people may need to take insulin.

Stroke

High blood pressure, elevated cholesterol, and diabetes all increase the risk of stroke. Therefore, it is not surprising that studies found higher rates of stroke in patients with schizophrenia. Although older age is a strong independent risk factor for stroke, one study found that younger people with schizophrenia (younger than 45 years old) were also at an increased risk of stroke.

Infectious Diseases

Infection with HIV (human immunodeficiency virus) is more common in people with schizophrenia than in the general population, with some studies reporting up to eight times higher infection rates. Human immunodeficiency virus is a retrovirus that causes acquired immunodeficiency syndrome (AIDS). HIV weakens the immune system, making the person more susceptible to infections and cancers, including life-threatening ones. Treatment consists of highly active antiretroviral therapy (HAART).

Rates of hepatitis B and hepatitis C infection are five to eleven times higher in people who have schizophrenia than in the general public. Hepatitis C is a chronic liver infection, which may lead to cirrhosis and hepatic failure (chronic liver damage and liver failure). Hepatitis B is primarily a short-lived infection of the liver that causes nausea, abdominal pain, fever, and jaundice (when the white of the eyes turn yellow). Both infections are spread through contact with infected blood and bodily fluids. The higher rates of these infectious diseases in people with schizophrenia is due primarily to higher intravenous drug use and unprotected sexual intercourse among these individuals.

Prevention of HIV and hepatitis B and C hinges on avoiding activities that carry a risk of becoming infected. For example, avoiding having unprotected intercourse and, for IV drug users, not sharing needles. Anyone with high-risk behaviors should undergo lab testing for these infections. Further, everyone between the ages of 15 and 65 should be screened for HIV, and everyone born between 1946 and 1965 should be tested for the hepatitis C antibody. Of the three infections, a vaccine exists only for hepatitis B. Anyone engaging in unsafe sex practices or sharing drug paraphernalia should receive this vaccine. The vaccine is also recommended for any sexually active person who is not in a long-term monogamous relationship and for men who have sex with men.

Cancer

Like heart disease, cancer is a significant contributor to the higher mortality rates in schizophrenia. While some studies have found conflicting results, there is evidence of an increased risk of lung and breast cancer. The increased risk of lung cancer is most closely linked to smoking cigarettes, which is common in people with schizophrenia. Cancers that develop at an older age, such as prostate, stomach, and pancreatic, may be less common in schizophrenia. In contrast, cancers with a younger age of onset (breast, uterine) may be more common.

A review of thirteen studies concluded that rates of breast cancer were higher in people with schizophrenia, though not all the studies reported increased rates. Risk factors for breast cancer in people with schizophrenia include obesity; low rates of screening with mammography; less breastfeeding; cigarette smoking; alcohol use; and lack of exercise. A higher incidence of lung cancer has been described in people who have schizophrenia, though many studies did not account for smoking, which may have been the key factor leading to higher rates.

Your loved one may not have received all the recommended cancer screening. Everyone should receive age-appropriate and risk-appropriate screening for common cancers (see table 7.1). People with schizophrenia and their families should talk to their health care providers about obtaining age-appropriate cancer screening. Colorectal cancer screening, typically with a colonoscopy, begins at age 50. Mammography is recommended for women starting at age 50. People aged 55 to 80 who currently smoke or recently quit should receive a chest CT scan to screen for lung cancer.

Support the Physical Health of Your Family Member

People with schizophrenia and their families must work with their mental health and medical care providers to better ensure screening for and treatment of common medical conditions. Evaluation of family and medical history, baseline weight and body mass index,

Table 7.1 Screening Recommendations for Selected Cancers (Abbreviated)

Breast cancer	Screening mammography for women aged 50–74 every 2 years
Colorectal cancer	Annual screening using fecal occult blood testing, sigmoidoscopy every 3–5 years, or colonoscopy every 10 years in adults beginning at age 50, continuing until age 75
Cervical cancer	Screening in women aged 21–65 with Pap smear every three years or in women aged 30–65 with a combination of Pap and human papillomavirus testing every 5 years
Prostate cancer	Screening with the PSA blood test not recommended
Lung cancer	Onetime low-dose computed tomography of the chest for men and women aged 55–80 who have a 30-pack/year smoking history and who currently smoke or have quit within the past 15 years.
Testicular cancer	Screening not recommended
Ovarian cancer	Screening not recommended
Pancreatic cancer	Screening not recommended

Source: United States Preventive Services Task Force, "Recommendations for Primary Care Practice," accessed March 28, 2015, www.uspreventiveservicestaskforce.org/Page/Name/recommendations.

blood pressure, fasting blood sugar, and lipid profiles should be assessed and followed appropriately by your family member's psychiatrist. You can support and encourage your loved one to exercise regularly and follow a diet low in fat and calories and high in fiber and lean protein. The individual, supported by family, should work with his psychiatrist to quit smoking or at a minimum to reduce the number of cigarettes smoked daily. His doctor should also assess sexual behaviors and counsel him as needed to reduce risk factors for contracting sexually transmitted infections.

Table 7.2 Metabolic Monitoring Guidelines for Patients on Antipsychotic Therapy

	Baseline	4 weeks	8 weeks	12 weeks	Every 3 months	Every year	Every 5 years
Personal/family	X					X	
Weight (BMI)	X	X	X	X	X		
Waist circumference	X					X	
Blood pressure	X			X		X	
Fasting blood glucose	X			X		X	
Fasting lipid profile	X			X			X

Source: Based on joint guidelines of the American Psychiatric Association and the American Diabetes Association. See American Diabetes Association, American Psychiatric Association, American Association of Clinical Endocrinologists, et al. "Consensus Development Conference on Antipsychotic Drugs and Obesity and Diabetes." *Diabetes Care* 27 (2004): 596–601.

Medication Side Effects

People who are being treated with antipsychotics are more likely to gain weight and have elevated cholesterol and sugar levels. Numerous studies have demonstrated this association, leading the U.S. Food and Drug Administration (FDA) to issue a warning about this entire class of medications. Certain medications, however, are more closely associated with these effects than others are. Weight gain occurs predominantly during the first few months of treatment, though it often continues at a slower pace for up to a year. The cause of this side effect is poorly understood. People who are normal weight before taking medication are more likely to gain weight, as are those who are taking antipsychotics for the first time.

The American Psychiatric Association and the American Diabetes Association issued joint guidelines for regular, systematic screening and monitoring of weight, cholesterol, blood sugar, blood pressure, and waist circumference for patients treated with antipsychotics (see table 7.2). The authors of this report also emphasized that the risk of weight gain, elevated cholesterol, and elevated blood sugar were different with each of the different antipsychotics. The highest risk agents are clozapine and olanzapine; risperidone and quetiapine pose an intermediate risk; and aripiprazole and ziprasidone have the lowest risk. Since these guidelines were issued, several new antipsychotics have become available. Among the newer agents, the greatest risk of weight gain is associated with asenapine (Saphris), followed by iloperidone (Fanapt) and paliperidone (Invega), with the lowest risk associated with lurasidone (Latuda) and lumateperone (Caplyta). Mental health care providers should be proactive about monitoring their patients' weight and ordering the appropriate monitoring blood tests. People with schizophrenia and their families should ask their mental health care providers whether all the appropriate screening tests for elevated blood sugar and elevated cholesterol have been completed, and what the results mean.

Managing Weight Gain

Several nonmedication approaches have been studied to help individuals lose weight and implement healthier lifestyles. Cognitive behavioral therapy (CBT) and nutrition counseling combined with exercise have been found effective. Group and individual counseling are beneficial for weight loss, but access to these services is limited by lack of insurance coverage and relatively few qualified providers trained in these specific counseling techniques. Nonetheless, general principles of healthy eating apply to everyone:

- Reduce portion size.
- Cut back on fast food and other restaurant food.
- Reduce your intake of soft drinks.
- Eat multiple small meals throughout the day.
- Do not skip breakfast.
- Eat more fruits and vegetables.

- Avoid excess intake of high-carbohydrate foods such as pasta, bread, and potatoes.

Another option is to switch to a different antipsychotic medication. Several studies have demonstrated weight loss associated with switching from one medication to another. For example, switching from olanzapine or risperidone to ziprasidone or aripiprazole may result in meaningful weight loss and improvement in blood sugar and cholesterol levels. Although this strategy is important to consider, people with schizophrenia and their psychiatrists should also take into account the stability that the current medication may be providing for treatment of psychiatric symptoms.

Various medications may be helpful for treating antipsychotic-induced weight gain. Note that none of the treatments discussed in this section is FDA approved for this particular use. The best-studied medication is metformin, which is a first-line treatment for diabetes mellitus. It is associated with weight loss and may both prevent and reverse weight gain due to antipsychotics. Nine clinical trials of metformin compared to placebo (sugar pill) have demonstrated its usefulness for weight loss. Most of the studies examined its use in individuals with schizophrenia who had gained a significant amount of weight after taking the antipsychotic medication olanzapine. In many studies metformin was combined with nutrition education and counseling.

In a review of seven well-designed studies, including nearly four hundred patients, metformin was associated with a 5 percent reduction in body weight (8 pounds on average). The most common adverse effects associated with metformin included gastrointestinal upset and diarrhea. A smaller number of studies found it to be useful when begun at the same time as the antipsychotic medication for prevention of weight gain. Topiramate is a seizure medication that may help with antipsychotic-induced weight gain, though less research supports its use.

Important Points
- People with schizophrenia have high rates of medical illness, particularly high blood pressure, obesity, elevated cholesterol, and diabetes.
- Death rates from heart disease are higher in schizophrenia. On average, a person with schizophrenia dies fifteen years earlier than those without the illness.
- Problems with access to and quality of medical care, dietary and lifestyle habits, and adverse effects of medication are among the factors that contribute to illness and death in people who have schizophrenia.
- Family members can be proactive in their loved one's medical care. This may mean assisting with medical appointments, communicating with primary care medical providers, and helping to schedule and complete recommended screening procedures.
- Help support your relative to lead a healthier lifestyle. This may include encouraging exercise or helping your loved one to eat more fruits and vegetables and avoid fast food and soft drinks.

Resources
American Diabetes Association, American Psychiatric Association, American Association of Clinical Endocrinologists, et al. "Consensus Development Conference on Antipsychotic Drugs and Obesity and Diabetes." *Diabetes Care* 27 (2004): 596–601.

Centers for Disease Control and Prevention. "Immunization Schedules for Adults in Easy-to-read Formats." Last updated February 12, 2020. www.cdc.gov/vaccines/schedules/easy-to-read/adult.html. A list of recommended vaccinations for adults.

National Institutes of Health. "Health Screening." *MedlinePlus.* National Library of Medicine. Last updated November 19, 2021. www.nlm.nih.gov

/medlineplus/healthscreening.html#summary. National Institutes of Health website summarizing recommended screening tests.

U.S. Preventive Services Task Force. www.uspreventiveservicestaskforce.org. Current screening procedures recommended by the United States Preventive Services Task Force.

Conclusion:
Looking to the Future

In this book we describe how medicine currently understands the causes and course of schizophrenia, as well as how we currently advise and treat people who have this disorder. We include family members and friends in the conversation because these individuals are so important in supporting and helping their loved one who has schizophrenia.

In closing we want to offer a glimpse into research now in progress to improve our understanding and treatment of schizophrenia. From the cause to the cure, medical and scientific researchers and clinicians are working hard to make discoveries that will make a difference.

The Causes of Schizophrenia

The cause of schizophrenia remains uncertain. It is clear, however, that disruption in brain development and function plays a crucial role in determining when it starts, how severe it is, and what course it takes. Efforts to understand what causes schizophrenia focus on a person's genetic makeup; structural and functional changes in the brain that can be assessed with imaging scans; other biological phenomena (such as inflammation, immune processes, and cortisol activity); and the role of environmental stressors. The potential value of these multifactorial investigations is supported by recent evidence indicating that variations in some of these "biological markers" may be more helpful in diagnosing and treating individuals than our present symptom-based approach.[1]

Stage-Related Treatment Approaches

Treatment of schizophrenia increasingly focuses on the specific phase of illness—that is, whether the person is at high risk, is experiencing a first episode, is early in the course of the illness, or is experiencing more chronic recurrent symptoms. In particular, efforts are ongoing to develop criteria that can help identify the illness as early as possible. One example is a recent pilot study that used computers to conduct an automated speech analysis of high-risk individuals.[2] Remarkably, the investigators were able to predict the later onset of psychosis with 100 percent accuracy. The hope is that approaches such as this will allow earlier recognition of schizophrenia and lead to treatment interventions that prevent the development of a more severe, recurrent form of the illness.

Another example of stage-related research is the NIMH Recovery After an Initial Schizophrenia Episode Early Treatment Program (RAISE ETP).[3] This controlled study employed a system of patient-centered, integrated treatment for first-episode psychosis called NAVIGATE. This involved coordinating a community care program that included optimized medication management, individual resiliency training, family education, and supported employment. After two years, the results were very encouraging, indicating that such interventions may favorably alter the illness's future course, especially in individuals who have a shorter duration of untreated psychosis.

If the person's symptoms reach a sustained stage, then treatment initially focuses on achieving response, to help the person remain in the community and avoid hospitalizations. When response is accomplished, the focus then shifts to achieving remission, which is characterized by few or no active symptoms. To the extent that remission can be accomplished, the chances of recovery are increased, allowing people with schizophrenia to function better and experience more satisfaction from life's activities. The ultimate aim is to improve quality of life and to provide the opportunity for people to achieve their personal goals. An important aspect of this process is the need to pay careful attention to medical problems, such as diabetes and heart disease, which occur more frequently in people with schizophrenia than in the general population, in part because of side effects associated with antipsychotics.[4] Chapter 7 covers this issue in more detail.

While antipsychotic medications remain an indispensable component of treatment, their benefits can be substantially enhanced by educational, social, psychological, and rehabilitative therapies, such as those described in chapter 4. Further, involving family and other support systems in these therapies to the extent possible can improve overall outcome. Thus, integrating biological and psychological therapies, as well actively involving important others in the person's life, are critical at all stages of this illness.

Treatment Adherence

People who have schizophrenia will do much better if they take their prescribed medications, and take them on schedule. Unfortunately, obstacles, many of them beyond anyone's control, can compromise even the best laid plans. To compensate for these problems and help with adherence, various strategies are available, such as the use of long-acting injectable (LAI) medication formulations.

More recent advances in technology are leading to novel ways to help with adherence. One example is an antipsychotic formulation containing an ingestible sensor.[5] When the medication comes in contact with the contents of the gastrointestinal tract, it sends a signal to another sensor located in a skin patch. In turn, this sensor provides information through a mobile phone to the person's caregivers, relating data about medication use, side effects, and possible worsening of symptoms. This tracking system not only improves monitoring of adherence, it also helps care providers to recognize and correct problems quickly so that treatment can continue. Such a digital health feedback system is currently approved by the FDA.

Another approach uses a mobile phone application (FOCUS) to help individuals manage their illness through a behavioral sensing system that quickly detects a worsening of symptoms.[6] This program also engages social workers, who send daily text messages to assess medication adherence as well as the person's overall state of health.

Treatment Resistance

Even when the optimal approach with presently available therapies is achieved, it may not be sufficient to adequately control all symptoms. In addition, there may be significant safety or tolerability issues, which make it impossible to achieve the maximum benefit. As a result, there are many ongoing attempts to develop newer, more effective, and safer therapies. These treatments can serve as alternatives to existing treatments or can be used in combination with existing treatments to improve the benefit and/or diminish side effects. Chapter 3 describes some of these therapies in more detail.

New Medication Strategies

One approach seeks to develop more effective medications based on our present knowledge about certain neurotransmitters, chemicals that facilitate communication between cells in brain areas thought to modulate the activities disrupted in schizophrenia. These new medications include drugs that alter the activity of dopamine, serotonin, glutamate, gamma-aminobutyric acid, acetylcholine, histamine, and other neurotransmitters in ways that differ from currently available medications.

A second approach is to repurpose medications originally developed for another illness but subsequently found to possibly help symptoms of schizophrenia. Two examples with early promise include the antibiotic minocycline (Dynacin), which may also be useful in the early stages of schizophrenia, and the antidepressant mirtazapine (Remeron).[7] Similarly, nutraceuticals such as omega-3 fatty acids, folate, and vitamin D have demonstrated potential benefit as preventive or early treatment strategies in preliminary studies. Finally, drugs with anti-inflammatory properties (such as aspirin); those that block the receptors mediating the effects of marijuana (such as cannabidiol); and those that work through hormonal mechanisms (such as cortisol, estrogen, or oxytocin) have also shown promise as add-on therapies.

Therapeutic Neuromodulation

The use of devices that alter the electrical activity of the brain may also play a supportive role when used with standard treatments. The earliest example is electroconvulsive therapy (ECT), developed to manage severe mood and psychotic symptoms over eighty years ago. Because of its side effects, however, its use is very limited at this time. Better tolerated approaches, such as transcranial magnetic stimulation (TMS) and transcranial direct stimulation (tDCS), are being studied as alternatives.[8]

Summary

Schizophrenia is a chronic illness that affects a person's thoughts, feelings, and behaviors. In particular, the ability to think clearly and to accurately interpret life experiences can be impaired by schizophrenia. This impairment leads to difficulties in relationships, in supporting and caring for oneself, and in achieving a satisfactory quality of life. Schizophrenia usually becomes evident in adolescence and follows a course characterized by periodic flare-ups and ongoing residual symptoms.

Although schizophrenia is a serious and debilitating illness, there is much room for optimism because of what medical and scientific researchers are learning about its causes. This increased understanding of cause can in turn improve the use of present treatments and guide the development of newer therapies, many of which are already on the horizon. An important aspect of this process is the need for people who have schizophrenia, their families, and treatment professionals to continue their efforts to advocate for the necessary resources so that the best care possible is delivered in the most appropriate settings.

Notes

Chapter 2. What Causes Schizophrenia?

1. J. van Os and S. Kapur, "Schizophrenia," *Lancet* 374 (2009): 635-45.
2. L. Arseneault et al., "Cannabis Use in Adolescence and Risk for Adult Psychosis: Longitudinal Prospective Study," *British Medical Journal* 325 (2002): 1212-13.
3. B. Moghaddam and D. Javitt, "From Revolution to Evolution: The Glutamate Hypothesis of Schizophrenia and Its Implication for Treatment," *Neuropsychopharmacology* 37, no. 1 (2012): 4-15; R. Y. Cho, R. O. Konecky, and C. S. Carter, "Impairments in Frontal Cortical Gamma Synchrony and Cognitive Control in Schizophrenia," *Proceedings of the National Academy of Science USA* 103, no. 52 (2006): 19878-83; O. D. Howes et al., "The Nature of Dopamine Dysfunction in Schizophrenia and What This Means for Treatment," *Archives of General Psychiatry* 69, no. 8 (2012): 776-86.
4. Arun K. Tiwari et al., "Genetics in Schizophrenia: Where Are We and What Next?" *Dialogues in Clinical Neuroscience* 12 (2010): 289-303.
5. F. Ferrarelli, "Endophenotypes and Biological Markers of Schizophrenia: From Biological Signs of Illness to Novel Treatment Targets," *Current Pharmaceutical Design* 19, no. 36 (2013): 6462-79.
6. Alan R. Sanders, "Genetics of Schizophrenia," in *Schizophrenia: Recent Advances in Diagnosis and Treatment*, ed. P. G. Janicak, S. Marder, R. Tandon, and M. Goldman, 139-60 (New York: Springer, 2014).
7. Schizophrenia Working Group of the Psychiatric Genomics Consortium, "Biological Insights from 108 Schizophrenia-Associated Genetic Loci," *Nature* 511 (2014): 421-27.
8. A. Sekar et al. "Schizophrenia Risk from Complex Variation of Complement Component 4." *Nature* 530 (2016): 177-83.

9. Cross-Disorder Group of the Psychiatric Genomics Consortium, "Identification of Risk Loci with Shared Effects on Five Major Psychiatric Disorders: A Genome-Wide Analysis," *Lancet* 381, no. 9875 (2013): 1371-79.

10. K. C. Murphy, L. A. Jones, and M. J. Owen, "High Rates of Schizophrenia in Adults with Velo-Cardio-Facial Syndrome," *Archives of General Psychiatry* 56 (1999): 616-22.

11. L. Wang, H. L. McLeod, and R. M. Weinshilbourn, "Genomics and Drug Response," *New England Journal of Medicine* 364, no. 12 (2011): 1144-53.

12. W. Pettersson-Yeo et al., "Dysconnectivity in Schizophrenia: Where Are We Now?" *Neuroscience and Behavioral Reviews* 35, no. 5 (2011): 1110-24.

Chapter 3. Biological Therapies for Schizophrenia

1. S. Ruhrmann et al., "Prediction of Psychosis in Adolescents and Young Adults at High Risk: Results from the Prospective European Prediction of Psychosis Study," *Archives of General Psychiatry* 67, no. 3 (2010): 241-51.

2. L. J. Seidman et al., "Neuropsychology of the Prodrome to Psychosis in the NAPLS Consortium: Relationship to Family History and Conversion to Psychosis," *Archives of General Psychiatry* 67, no. 6 (2010): 578-88.

3. A. Preti and M. Cella, "Randomized-Controlled Trials in People at Ultra High Risk of Psychosis: A Review of Treatment Effectiveness," *Schizophrenia Research* 123, no. 1 (2010): 30-36; P. D. McGorry et al., "Intervention in Individuals at Ultra-High Risk for Psychosis: A Review and Future Directions," *Journal of Clinical Psychiatry* 70, no. 9 (2009): 1206-12.

4. G. P. Amminger et al., "Long-Chain Omega-3 Fatty Acids for Indicated Prevention of Psychotic Disorders: A Randomized, Placebo-Controlled Trial," *Archives of General Psychiatry* 67, no. 2 (2010): 146-54.

5. P. D. McGorry et al., "Randomized Controlled Trial of Interventions Designed to Reduce the Risk of Progression to First-Episode Psychosis in a Clinical Sample with Subthreshold Symptoms," *Archives of General Psychiatry* 59, no. 10 (2002): 921-28.

6. M. J. Cuesta et al., "Duration of Untreated Negative and Positive Symptoms of Psychosis and Cognitive Impairment in First Episode Psychosis," *Schizophrenia Research* 141, no. 2-3 (2012): 222-27.

7. M. Bertelsen et al., "Five-Year Follow-Up of a Randomized Multicenter Trial of Intensive Early Intervention vs. Standard Treatment for Patients with a First Episode of Psychotic Illness: The OPUS Trial," *Archives of General Psychiatry* 65, no. 7 (2008): 762-71; W. ten Velden Hegelstad et al., "Long-Term Follow-Up of the TIPS Early Detection in Psychosis Study: Effects on 10-Year Outcome," *American Journal of Psychiatry* 169 (2012): 374-80; L. Wunderink et al., "Recovery in Remitted First-Episode Psychosis at 7 Years of Follow-Up of an Early Dose Reduction/Discon-

tinuation or Maintenance Treatment Strategy: Long-Term Follow-Up of a 2-Year Randomized Clinical Trial," *Journal of the American Medical Association Psychiatry*, published electronically July 3, 2013.

8. P. G. Janicak, S. Marder, and M. Pavuluri, *Principles and Practice of Psychopharmacotherapy*, 5th ed. (Philadelphia, PA: Lippincott Williams and Wilkins, 2011), 77-180.

9. S. Leucht et al., "Comparative Efficacy and Tolerability of 15 Antipsychotic Drugs in Schizophrenia: A Multiple-Treatments Meta-Analysis," *Lancet* 382, no. 9896 (2013): 951-62; C. Schneider, R. Corrigall, D. Hayes, M. Kyriakopoulos, and S. Frangou, "Systematic Review of the Efficacy and Tolerability of Clozapine in the Treatment of Youth with Early Onset Schizophrenia," *European Psychiatry*, published electronically October 9, 2013.

10. L. Citrome, "Inhaled Loxapine for Agitation," *Current Psychiatry* 12, no. 2 (2013): 31-36.

11. P. G. Janicak, S. M. Dowd, J. T. Rado, and M. J. Welch, "The Re-Emerging Role of Therapeutic Neuromodulation," *Current Psychiatry* 9, no. 11 (2010): 67-74.

12. P. G. Janicak and K. Hussain, "Drug-Induced Movement Disorders," in *Comprehensive Textbook of Psychiatry*, vol. 2, 10th ed., ed. B. J. Sadock, V. A. Sadock, P. Ruiz (Philadelphia, PA: Lippincott Williams and Wilkins, in press).

13. C. Das, G. Mendez, S. Jagasia, and L. A. Labbate, "Second-Generation Antipsychotic Use in Schizophrenia and Associated Weight Gain: A Critical Review and Meta-Analysis of Behavioral and Pharmacologic Treatments," *Annals of Clinical Psychiatry* 24, no. 3 (2012): 225-39.

Chapter 4. Psychosocial and Behavioral Treatments for Schizophrenia

1. J. Sin and I. Norman, "Psychoeducational Interventions for Family Members of People with Schizophrenia: A Mixed-Method Systematic Review," *Journal of Clinical Psychiatry* 74, no. 12 (2013): e1145-62.

2. A. Lucksted, W. McFarlane, D. Downing, L. Dixon, and C. Adams, "Recent Developments in Family Psychoeducation as an Evidence-Based Practice," *Journal Marital Family Therapy* 38, no. 1 (2012): 101-21.

3. J. Xia, L. B. Merinder, and M. R. Belgamwar, "Psychoeducation for Schizophrenia," *Cochrane Database Systematic Reviews* 6 (2011): CD002831; C. Rummel-Kluge and W. Kissling, "Psychoeducation for Patients with Schizophrenia and Their Families," *Expert Review of Neurotherapeutics* 8, no. 7 (2008): 1067-77.

4. K. T. Mueser, F. Deavers, D. L. Penn, and J. E. Cassisi, "Psychosocial Treatments for Schizophrenia," *Annual Review of Clinical Psychology* 9 (2013): 465-97.

5. R. S. Kern et al., "Psychosocial Rehabilitation and Psychotherapy Approaches," in *Schizophrenia: Recent Advances in Diagnosis and Treatment*, ed. P. G. Janicak, S. R. Marder, R. Tandon, and M. Goldman, 139-60 (New York: Springer, 2014).

6. Ibid.

7. S. J. Ziguras and G. W. Stuart, "A Meta-analysis of the Effectiveness of Mental Health Case Management over 20 Years," *Psychiatric Services* 51 (2000): 1410-21.

8. G. R. Bond, R. E. Drake, and D. R. Becker, "An Update on Randomized Controlled Trials for Evidence Based Supported Employment," *Psychiatric Rehabilitation Journal* 31 (2008): 280-90.

9. T. Marshall, R. W. Goldberg, L. Braude, et al., "Supported Employment: Assessing the Evidence," *Psychiatric Services* 65 (2014): 16-23.

10. A. Medalia and J. Choi, "Cognitive Remediation in Schizophrenia," *Neuropsychology Review* 19 (2009): 353-64.

11. M. Fisher, C. Holland, K. Subramaniam, and S. Vinogradov, "Neuroplasticity-Based Cognitive Training in Schizophrenia: An Interim Report on the Effects 6 Months Later," *Schizophrenia Bulletin* 36 (2010): 869-79.

12. T. Wykes, V. Huddy, C. Cellard, S. R. McGurk, and P. Czobor, "A Meta-analysis of Cognitive Remediation for Schizophrenia: Methodology and Effect Sizes," *American Journal of Psychiatry* 168 (2011): 472-85; K. Subramaniam, T. L. Luks, M. Fisher, et al., "Computerized Cognitive Training Restores Neural Activity within the Reality Monitoring Network in Schizophrenia," *Neuron* 23 (2012): 842-53.

13. A. Medalia and A. M. Saperstein, "Does Cognitive Remediation for Schizophrenia Improve Functional Outcomes?" *Current Opinion in Psychiatry* 26 (2013): 151-57.

14. M. D. Bell, K. H. Choi, C. Dyer, and B. E. Wexler, "Benefits of Cognitive Remediation and Supported Employment for Schizophrenia Patients with Poor Community Functioning," *Psychiatric Services*, published electronically January 2, 2014.

15. S. Mead, D. Hilton, and L. Curtis, "Peer Support: A Theoretical Perspective," *Psychiatric Rehabilitation Journal* 25 (2001): 134-41.

16. S. Murphy, C. B. Irving, C. E. Adams, and R. Driver, "Crisis Intervention for People with Severe Mental Illness," *Cochrane Database Systematic Reviews* 16, no. 5 (2012): CD001087; W. H. Sledge, M. Lawless, D. Sells, et al., "Effectiveness of Peer Support in Reducing Readmissions of Persons with Multiple Psychiatric Hospitalizations," *Psychiatric Services* 62 (2011): 541-44; J. A. Cook, P. Steigman, S. Pickett, et al., "Randomized Controlled Trial of Peer-Led Recovery Education Using Building Recovery of

Individual Dreams and Goals through Education and Support (BRIDGES)," *Schizophrenia Research* 136 (2012): 36-42.

17. J. M. Hooley, "Expressed Emotion and Relapse of Psychopathology," *Annual Review of Clinical Psychology* 3 (2007): 329-52.

18. J. D. Prince, "Family Involvement and Satisfaction with Community Mental Health Care of Individuals with Schizophrenia," *Community Mental Health Journal* 41 (2005): 419-30.

19. F. Pharoah, J. Mari, J. Rathbone, and W. Wong, "Family Intervention for Schizophrenia," *Cochrane Database Systematic Reviews*, no. 12, published electronically December 8, 2010, CD000088.

20. G. Dunn, D. Fowler, R. Rollinson, et al., "Effective Elements of Cognitive Behavior Therapy for Psychosis: Results of a Novel Type of Subgroup Analysis Based on Principal Stratification," *Psychological Medicine* 42 (2012): 1057-68.

21. P. M. Grant, G. A. Huh, D. Perivoliotis, N. M. Stolar, and A. T. Beck, "Randomized Trial to Evaluate the Efficacy of Cognitive Therapy for Low-Functioning Patients with Schizophrenia," *Archives of General Psychiatry* 69 (2012): 121-27; S. Klingberg, W. Wolwer, C. Engel, et al., "Negative Symptoms of Schizophrenia as Primary Target of Cognitive Behavioral Therapy: Results of the Randomized Clinical TONES Study," *Schizophrenia Bulletin* 37, no. S37 (2011): S98-110; A. Bechdolf, B. Knost, B. Nelson, et al., "Randomized Comparison of Group Cognitive Behavior Therapy and Group Psychoeducation in Acute Patients with Schizophrenia: Effects on Subjective Quality of Life," *Australia and New Zealand Journal of Psychiatry* 44, no. 2 (2010): 144-50.

22. F. Sarin, L. Wallin, and B. Widerlov, "Cognitive Behavior Therapy for Schizophrenia: A Meta-analytical Review of Randomized Controlled Trials," *Nordic Journal of Psychiatry* 65 (2011): 162-74; P. Hutton and P. J. Taylor, "Cognitive Behavioral Therapy for Psychosis Prevention: A Systematic Review and Meta-analysis," *Psychological Medicine* 44, no. 3 (2014): 449-68; J. Addington, C. Marshall, and P. French, "Cognitive Behavioral Therapy in Prodromal Psychosis," *Current Pharmaceutical Design* 18 (2012): 558-65.

23. D. Turkington, T. Sensky, J. Scott, et al., "A Randomized Controlled Trial of Cognitive-Behavior Therapy for Persistent Symptoms in Schizophrenia: A Five-Year Follow-Up," *Schizophrenia Research* 98, no. 1-3 (2008): 1-7.

24. M. Schulz, R. Gray, A. Spiekermann, C. Abderhalden, J. Behrens, and M. Driessen, "Adherence Therapy Following an Acute Episode of Schizophrenia: A Multi-centre Randomized Controlled Trial," *Schizophrenia Research* 146, no. 1-3 (2013): 59-63.

25. P. M. Grant, J. Reisweber, L. Luther, A. P. Brinen, and A. T. Beck, "Successfully Breaking a 20-Year Cycle of Hospitalizations with Recovery Oriented Cognitive Therapy for Schizophrenia," *Psychological Services,* published electronically September 30, 2013.

26. S. Dowd and P. G. Janicak, *Integrating Psychological and Biological Therapies in Clinical Practice* (Philadelphia, PA: Lippincott Williams and Wilkins, 2009).

Conclusion: Looking to the Future

1. B. Clementz, J. Sweeney, J. Hamm, et al., "Identification of Distinct Psychosis Biotypes Using Brain-Based Biomarkers," *American Journal Psychiatry,* published electronically September 18, 2015.

2. G. Bedi, F. Carrillo, G. A. Cecchi, et al., "Automated Analysis of Free Speech Predicts Psychosis Onset in High-Risk Youths," *npj Schizophrenia* 1 (2015): article number 15030.

3. J. Kane, D. Robinson, N. Schooler, et al. "Comprehensive versus Usual Community Care for First-Episode Psychosis: 2 Year Outcomes from the NIMH RAISE Early Treatment Program," *American Journal of Psychiatry,* published electronically September 4, 2015.

4. C. Green, B. Yarborough, M. Leo, et al., "The STRIDE Weight Loss and Lifestyle Intervention for Individuals Taking Antipsychotic Medications: A Randomized Trial," *American Journal of Psychiatry* 172, no. 1 (2015): 71–81.

5. J. Kane, R. Perlis, L. DiCarlo, et al., "First Experience with a Wireless System Incorporating Physiological Assessments and Direct Confirmation of Digital Tablet Ingestions in Ambulatory Patients with Schizophrenia or Bipolar Disorder," *Journal of Clinical Psychiatry* 74, no. 6 (2013): e533–e540.

6. D. Ben-Zeev, C. Brenner, M. Begale, et al., "Feasibility, Acceptability and Preliminary Evidence of a Smartphone Intervention for Schizophrenia," *Schizophrenia Bulletin* 40, no. 6 (2014): 1244–53.

7. D. Kelly, K. Sullivan, J. McEvoy, et al., "Adjunctive Minocycline in Clozapine-Treated Schizophrenia Patients with Persistent Symptoms," *Journal of Clinical Psychopharmacology* 35, no. 4 (2015): 374–78; F. Liu, X. Gao, R. Wu, et al., "Minocycline Supplementation for Treatment of Negative Symptoms in Early-Phase Schizophrenia: A Double Blind, Randomized, Controlled Trial," *Schizophrenia Research* 153, no. 1-3 (2014): 169–76; V. Terevnikov, G. Joffe, and J. H. Stenberg, "Randomized Controlled Trials of Add-On Antidepressants in Schizophrenia," *International Journal of Neuropsychopharmacology* 18, no. 9 (2015), published electronically May 19, 2015.

8. J. T. Rado and E. I. Hernandez, "Therapeutic Neuromodulation for Treatment of Schizophrenia," in *Schizophrenia: Recent Advances in Diagnosis and Treatment,* ed. P. G. Janicak, S. R. Marder, R. Tandon, and M. Goldman, 139–60 (New York: Springer, 2014).

Index

acceptance of illness, 72-73, 84

acetylcholine, 44, 112

adherence therapy, 61

adherence to treatment, 29, 38, 53-54, 63-68, 110-11; factors affecting, 53, 64-68, 71; family support of, 68, 73-74, 84-85; strategies to enhance, 66-67, 68, 110-11

adoption studies, 26

affect, flat or blunted, 3, 7

agranulocytosis, 51

akathisia, 40, 47, 65

akinesia, 65

alcohol use, 12, 17, 24, 49, 89, 90, 101

alogia, 7

alprazolam (Xanax), 17

Alzheimer's disease, 18

American Diabetes Association, 103

American Psychiatric Association (APA), 11, 103

amlodipine, 97

amphetamine salts (Adderall), 17

anger, 7, 10, 14, 16, 69, 88-89; of family, 83, 91

angiotensin-converting enzyme (ACE) inhibitors, 97

angiotensin receptor blockers, 97

anhedonia, 7, 13

antianxiety drugs, 17, 41

anticholinergic drugs, 41; side effects, 47, 48, 51

antidepressants, 41, 112

antihypertensive drugs, 97

anti-inflammatory drugs, 46, 112

antipsychotic drugs, 35-53, 110; for acute symptom management, 38-42, 46; Clinical Antipsychotic Trials of Intervention Effectiveness (CATIE) study of, 96, 97; dosing and formulations of, 39-40, 43-44; drug interactions with, 52; in early course of illness, 36, 38; first-generation, 39, 47; with ingestible sensor, 111; in later course of illness, 35, 38-42; long-acting injectable, 39, 40, 42-43, 44, 46, 68, 111; for long-term management, 35, 42-43; resistance to, 35, 43-46, 111-12; second-generation, 40, 48; switching between, 47, 49, 51, 52, 67, 105. *See also* adherence to treatment; *specific drugs*

antipsychotic drug side effects, 39, 46-53; anticholinergic, 51; cardiovascular, 50, 97; discontinuation due to, 65-66;

antipsychotic drug side effects (*cont.*)
extrapyramidal, 65; hematologic, 51;
monitoring for, 103-4; neurological,
47-49; prolactin, 50-51; sedative, 52;
weight and metabolic, 49-50, 103-5
antiretroviral therapy, 100
anxiety, 2, 10-11, 40
apathy, 7
aripiprazole (Abilify), 40, 48, 51, 104,
105
asenapine (Saphris), 40, 48, 104
aspirin, 46, 112
assertive community treatment (ACT),
57, 68
association studies, 26-27
attention deficit disorder, 17, 27
attention problems, 2, 9, 25, 32, 53, 58
avolition, 7

behavior, 2, 19; catatonic, 4, 11;
disorganized, 4, 8-9; family effects
of, 81
behavioral family therapy, 60
benzodiazepines, 17, 49
benztropine (Cogentin), 41, 65
biological markers, 25, 26, 28, 30, 109
biological therapies, 34-54; in early
course of illness, 35-38; in later course
of illness, 35, 38-42; for long-term
management, 35, 42-43; mechanisms
of action of, 29, 43, 44-45, 112; resistance to, 35, 43-46, 111-12; risks/side
effects of, 46-53; stage-related, 34-43,
109-10; therapeutic neuromodulation,
45, 52-53, 112
bipolar disorder, 2-3, 15, 16, 27
Bleuler, Eugen, 3
blood pressure: antipsychotic effects
on, 49, 50, 52; elevated, 42, 95, 96, 97,
98, 99, 106; ideal, 97; metabolic
syndrome and, 99; monitoring of,
102, 103

blood sugar: antipsychotic effects on,
49, 72, 96, 98, 99; monitoring of, 102,
103, 104
body dysmorphic disorder, 16
brain abnormalities, 1, 23-24, 31-33,
108-9; functional, 23-24; imaging of,
13, 20, 30-32, 109; structural, 23, 31-32
brain networks, 32
brain neuroplasticity, 59
brain neurotransmitters (NTs), 23-24,
25, 27, 44-45, 47, 51, 112
brain systems, 32
breast cancer, 101, 102
brexpiprazole (Rexulti), 40, 48
brief psychotic disorder, 14

calcium channel blockers, 97
cancer, 51, 94, 96, 100-101; screening for,
97, 101, 102
candidate gene association studies,
26, 39
Caplyta (lumateperone), 40, 104
cardiovascular side effects, 47, 48, 50, 97
cariprazine (Vraylar), 40, 48
causes/risk factors, 21-33, 36, 108-9; early
recognition of, 35-36, 37, 38; external
factors, 21-22; genetics, 21, 22, 24, 25-30;
interactions between, 24; internal
factors, 22-23; risk prediction, 28
celecoxib, 46
cervical cancer, 97, 102
chlorpromazine (Thorazine), 39, 47
chlorthalidone, 97
cholesterol, elevated, 49, 95, 96, 97-98,
99, 103, 104, 105, 106
Clinical Antipsychotic Trials of
Intervention Effectiveness (CATIE),
96, 97
clonazepam (Klonopin), 17
clozapine (Clozaril), 39-41, 48, 49, 51, 104
cocaine, 17
cognition-enhancing techniques, 58

cognitive behavioral therapy (CBT), 36-37, 60, 61-62, 104; for family, 88; for psychosis (CBTp), 61
cognitive impairment, 2, 9-10, 37
cognitive remediation (CR), 57, 58-59, 60
colorectal cancer, 97, 101, 102
communication, 8; cognitive deficits and, 9-10; in family, 77, 79-81
compensatory techniques, 58
computerized tomography (CT), 13, 30, 101
concentration problems, 2, 9, 19, 53, 69, 86
copy number variations, 28
cortisol, 24, 109, 112
course of illness, 2-3, 19, 25, 30, 108, 113; prediction of, 19, 30, 36; stage-related treatment during, 35-43, 109-10
crisis intervention, 59
cultural factors, 22, 26, 65

dangerousness, 1, 75, 87, 88-89
deep brain stimulation (DBS), 45, 52-53
de-escalation techniques, 40-41
definitions, 7-8; schizophrenia, 2-3
delirium, 18-19, 51
delusional disorder, 14
delusions, 2, 3, 4-6, 7, 19, 23; family response to, 79-80; in mania, 16; types of, 5-6; violence and, 88
dementia praecox, 2
denial of illness, 65, 72
depression, 2, 10, 12-13; major, 15-16; treatment of, 38
derailment, 8
diabetes mellitus, 42, 49, 72, 93, 94, 95-96, 98-99, 105, 106, 110; antipsychotic-induced, 41
diagnosis, 3-4, 20; criteria for, 12, 20, 109; early, importance of, 35-36, 37, 38; initial evaluation for, 11-13;

neuroimaging for, 13, 20, 30-32; vs. other psychiatric disorders, 15-16, 20
Diagnostic and Statistical Manual of Mental Disorders (DSM-5), 12
diffusion-weighted tension imaging (DTI), 30
diuretics, 97
donepezil, 49
dopamine, 23-24, 27, 32, 44, 47, 50, 112
drill-and-practice techniques, 59

early course of illness, 35-38
echopraxia, 11
ecstasy, 17
electroconvulsive therapy (ECT), 45, 52, 112
emotion, expressed (EE), 81
emotional expression, 2, 3, 7, 10-11, 23; in family, 60, 81, 87
employment, 1, 4, 8, 9, 16, 58, 84; of family member, 78, 82; medication use and, 64, 68; supported, 57, 58, 59
enalapril, 97
endophenotypes, 25
environmental stress, 21, 22, 24, 26, 33, 80, 109
epigenetics, 24
estrogen, 45, 51, 112
exercise, 70, 71, 72, 93, 97, 99, 101, 102, 106; cognitive, 58-59; for weight control, 98, 104
extrapyramidal side effects (EPS), 65

family, 2, 77-92; communication in, 77, 79-81; education for, 56, 60, 71, 78, 83-84, 109; expanding roles of, 77-78; expressed emotion in, 60, 81, 87; feelings of, 81-83; LEAP method for, 74, 76; maintaining routines of, 87; meeting needs of, 87; recognizing first signs of relapse, 69, 85-86; strategies for, 83-88; of suicidal

family (*cont.*)
person, 89-91; support for, 87-88; support of long-term recovery, 88; support of physical health of ill person, 101-2, 106; support of treatment adherence, 68, 73-74, 84-85; violence in, 88-89
family history, 25-26, 31, 36
family studies, 25-26
family therapy (FT), 60, 62, 88
"Family to Family" program, 84
fatigue, 52, 69; of family, 83, 91
fear, 1, 7, 10, 11, 69, 75, 89; of developing schizophrenia, 83
financial management, 9, 10, 57, 81, 83, 86
fluphenazine (Prolixin), 39, 47
FOCUS mobile phone app, 111
folate, 45, 112
free radicals, 23, 45
frustration of family, 73, 80, 81-82, 83, 84, 85, 91
functional impairment, 1, 2, 4, 8, 12, 16, 19, 37; after relapse, 64

gamma-aminobutyric acid, 23, 44, 112
gender factors, 4, 22, 50, 94, 98-99
genetics, 21, 22, 24, 25-30, 33, 36, 109; epidemiological, 25-26; epigenetics, 24; molecular, 26-28; pharmacogenetics and pharmacogenomics, 28-29, 39
genetic testing, 28
genome-wide association studies (GWAS), 27; cross-disorder analyses, 27-28
glutamate, 23, 27, 33, 44, 112
guilt, 90; delusions of, 6; of parents, 82

hallucinations, 1, 3, 4, 6, 8, 19, 23; auditory, 2, 3, 6, 38, 45, 70, 72, 73, 90; types of, 6; visual, 6, 17, 18

hallucinogens, 17
haloperidol (Haldol), 39, 47
health care, 96-97
heart disease, 93, 94-96, 97, 98, 99, 106, 110
hematologic side effects, 47, 48, 51
hepatitis B and C, 100
heroin, 17
histamine, 45, 112
HIV/AIDS, 99-100
hopelessness, 10, 67, 76, 81, 90
hormones, 24, 50, 99
hormone therapies, 45, 112
hospitalization, 6, 37, 38, 64, 65, 77-78
hydrochlorothiazide, 97
hyperlipidemia. *See* cholesterol, elevated
hypertension. *See* blood pressure: elevated
hypothalamic-pituitary-adrenal axis, 24

idea of reference (type of delusion), 5, 88
illness/wellness/recovery skills training, 57
iloperidone (Fanapt), 40, 48, 104
immune system, 24, 27, 109
independence of ill person, 19, 68; family encouragement of, 86, 87; skills training for, 57
infections, 13, 19, 24, 27, 99-100; clozapine and, 51; DBS-related, 53; hepatitis B and C, 100; HIV, 99-100; maternal, 21; sexually transmitted, 99-100, 102
information processing, 10, 58, 72, 79
inhalants, 17
insight into illness, 56, 59, 64, 67, 72-73, 76, 84

ketamine, 17
Kraepelin, Emil, 2

language problems, 9, 25
later course of illness, 35, 38-42
LEAP (listen, empathize, agree, and partner) method, 74, 76
life expectancy, 49, 94, 97, 106
linkage studies, 26
lisinopril, 97
long-acting injectable (LAI) medications, 39, 40, 42-43, 44, 46, 68, 111
long-term management, 35, 42-43
looseness of association, 8
lorazepam (Ativan), 17
losartan, 97
loss, feelings of, 82
loxapine (Adasuve, Loxitane), 39, 47
lumateperone (Caplyta), 40, 104
lung cancer, 100-101, 102
lurasidone (Latuda), 40, 48, 104
lysergic acid diethylamide (LSD), 17

magnetic resonance imaging (MRI), 13, 30
magnetic resonance spectroscopy (MRS), 31
mania, 14, 15-16
mannerisms, 11
marijuana, 17, 18, 22, 36, 49, 71, 112
medical conditions, 18-19, 93-106, 110; family support of physical health, 101-2, 106; health care for, 95-96; screening for, 96-97. *See also specific conditions*
medications, 34-54, 110; benefits and risks of, 34, 39, 46, 54; in early course of illness, 35-38; education about, 56; in later course of illness, 35, 38-42; for long-term management, 35, 42-43; mechanisms of action of, 29, 43, 44, 112; pharmacogenetics and pharmacogenomics of, 28-29, 39; predicting response to, 29, 39; repurposing of, 45-46, 112; resistance to, 35, 43-46, 111-12; side effects, 103-4; taking,

64-68. *See also* adherence to treatment; antipsychotic drugs
memory problems, 2, 18, 25, 32, 53, 58; antipsychotic-induced, 51; and working memory, 9, 31, 58
menstrual period, 50
mesoridazine (Serentil), 39, 47
metabolic side effects, 49-50, 99; monitoring for, 103-4
metabolic syndrome, 41, 98-99
metformin, 50, 99, 105
methylphenidate (Ritalin), 17
methylprednisolone, 18
minocycline (Dynacin), 112
mirtazapine (Remeron), 112
molindone (Moban), 39, 47
mood disorders, 15-16
mood symptoms, 2, 10-11, 12, 14, 19
motivation, lack of, 3, 7, 8
movement abnormalities, 2, 11; drug-induced, 40, 47-49, 65
multifamily group therapy, 60
mutism, 11
myelin, 23

narcotic pain medications, 17
National Alliance on Mental Illness (NAMI), 11, 71, 84
NAVIGATE strategy, 109
neologisms, 8
neuroimaging, 13, 20, 30-32, 109
neuroleptic malignant syndrome, 52
neurological side effects, 47-49
neuromodulation, therapeutic, 45, 52-53, 112
neurotransmitters (NTs), 23-24, 25, 27, 44-45, 47, 51, 112
nonsteroidal anti-inflammatory drugs (NSAIDs), 46
norepinephrine, 44
nutraceuticals, 36, 45, 46, 112
nutritional counseling, 50, 104, 105

nutritional deficiencies, 22, 24
nutrition/diet, 49, 50, 71, 72, 93, 97, 98, 99, 102, 106

obesity, 93, 94, 98, 101, 106. *See also* weight gain, drug-induced
obsessive-compulsive disorder, 16
olanzapine (Zyprexa), 40, 48, 97, 104, 105
omega-3 fatty acids, 36, 45, 46, 112
ovarian cancer, 102
oxytocin, 45, 112

paliperidone (Invega), 40, 42, 44, 48, 68, 104
pancreatic cancer, 101, 102
paranoia, 15, 36, 38, 70, 71, 72, 74, 84, 88
paranoid personality disorder, 14, 15
Parkinson's disease, 18, 47
peer interventions, 57, 59, 60
perceptual distortions, 3, 4-6, 8, 13-15, 17, 23
perinatal factors, 21-22
perphenazine (Trilafon), 39, 47
personality disorders, 14-15
pharmacogenetics and pharmacogenomics, 28-29, 39
phencyclidine (angel dust), 17
positron emission tomography (PET), 30
posttraumatic stress disorder, 16
prednisone, 18
problem-solving skills, 10, 56, 58
prolactin side effects, 47, 48, 50-51
prostate cancer, 101, 102
pseudoparkinsonism, 47
psilocybin, 17
Psychiatric Genomic Consortium, 28
psychoeducation, 34, 35, 36, 37, 38, 42, 46, 54, 55, 56, 110; for family, 56, 60, 71, 78, 83-84, 109
psychosis, 2, 7; drug-induced, 17-18; in medical conditions, 18-19; in mood

disorders, 16; in schizophrenia-spectrum disorders, 13-15
psychosocial and behavioral interventions, 55-62
psychosocial rehabilitation, 56-60, 61, 110
psychotherapy, 34, 35, 54, 55, 60-62

quality of life, 42, 55, 58, 110, 113
quetiapine (Seroquel), 40, 44, 48, 49, 97, 104

recovery, 37, 42, 57, 59, 62, 75; family support of, 85, 88
Recovery After an Initial Schizophrenia Episode Early Treatment Program (RAISE ETP), 109-10
recovery-oriented cognitive therapy, 62
referral to mental health care provider, 11
relapse, 63; family emotion and, 60, 81; first signs of, 69, 85-86; prevalence of, 64; substance abuse and, 71
relapse prevention, 69-72; cognitive behavioral therapy (CBT) for, 61; education for, 56; family therapy for, 60, 62, 88; medication adherence for, 29, 53, 63-68, 76; stress management for, 71-72
remission, 42, 64, 110
resistance to treatment, 35, 43-46, 111-12
risperidone (Risperdal), 36, 40, 44, 48, 97, 104, 105

sadness, 10, 15, 16, 88, 90; of family, 81, 83, 91
schizoaffective disorder, 14
schizoid personality disorder, 14, 15
schizophrenia-spectrum disorders, 13-15
schizophreniform disorder, 13-14
schizotypal personality disorder, 14-15
Schneider, Kurt, 3

school problems, 1, 4, 7, 8, 9, 10, 12, 13, 16, 76, 82; medication use and, 64, 68, 74
screening, medical, 96-97
sedation, drug-induced, 47, 48, 52
sedatives, 41
seizures, 19, 41, 52
serotonin, 33, 44, 112
sexual behavior, 100, 102
sexual side effects, 50
shame, feelings of, 75, 82, 91
skills training, 46, 57, 59, 61; for family, 88
sleep, 10, 41, 52, 65, 69, 71, 72, 86
smoking: cigarettes, 49, 94, 101, 102; marijuana, 18
social cognition, 10
social cognition training, 57
social interventions, 34, 35, 37, 42, 54, 55; psychosocial rehabilitation, 56-60, 61, 110
social skills training, 46, 57, 60, 61
social withdrawal, 2, 6, 7, 12-13
speech: disorganized, 4, 8; poverty of, 7
stage-related treatments, 34-43, 109-10; in early course of illness, 35-38; in later course of illness, 35, 38-42; long-term management, 35, 42-43
steroids, 18, 45
stigma, 63, 75-76, 82
stimulant drugs, 17
stomach cancer, 101
strengths of ill person, 86-87, 91
stress, 13, 22, 24, 86; abnormal response to, 23, 24; environmental, 21, 24, 26, 33, 80, 109; family coping/reduction of, 56, 84, 85, 87, 88; management of, 63, 71-72, 76; perinatal, 21-22; violence and, 88
stress-vulnerability models, 56
stroke, 99
substance use/abuse, 12, 17-18, 22, 36, 49, 89; treatment of, 38, 61

suicide, 37, 40, 89-91, 94
supported employment (SE), 57, 58, 59
support groups/programs, 37, 59, 68, 71
suspiciousness, 14-15, 36
symptoms, 1-2, 4-7, 9-11, 19; age at onset of, 2, 4, 13, 19; negative, 3, 4, 6-7, 8, 12-13, 19, 61, 81; positive, 4-6, 7, 61; triggers for, 13; variation of, 12, 19, 55

tangentiality, 8
tardive dyskinesia (TD), 49
testicular cancer, 102
thinking, disorganized, 8, 31, 66-67, 76
thioridazine (Mellaril), 39, 47
thiothixene (Navane), 39, 47
thought broadcasting, 3, 5
thought insertion, 3, 5
thought withdrawal, 3, 5
topiramate, 50, 105-6
transcranial direct cortical stimulation (tDCS), 45, 112
transcranial magnetic stimulation (TMS), 45, 52, 112
treatment(s): biological, 34-54; psychosocial and behavioral, 55-62; resistance to, 35, 43-46, 111-12; response to, 29, 30, 42, 110; stage-related, 34-43, 109-10. *See also* adherence to treatment
trifluoperazine (Stelazine), 39, 47
triglycerides, 49, 98
trust in mental health care provider, 65-66, 76, 85
twin studies, 26

uterine cancer, 101

valsartan, 97
verbal fluency, 9
violence, 1, 87, 88-89
vitamin B6, 49
vitamin D, 45, 112

weight gain, drug-induced, 41, 47, 48, 49-50, 98; management of, 104-5; monitoring for, 103-4

wellness maintenance, 63-76; acceptance of illness, 63, 72-73; family role in, 73-74, 76; recognizing first signs of relapse, 69, 85-86; relapse prevention, 69-72; stigma and, 63, 75-76; stress management, 71-72; treatment adherence for, 64-68, 76

word salad, 8

working alliance, 37, 53

ziprasidone (Geodon), 40, 48, 105